NEW OFFER
Online Study Secrets Course!

Dear Customer,

Struggle with tests? Short on time? Not sure where to even *start* studying? Mometrix has designed a new Study Secrets Course to help every student, no matter what study scenario you are in.

This online course guides you through the full process, from study preparation to test day, so you'll be ready to ace your next exam. The Study Secrets Course contains **14 in-depth lessons** that break down top study strategies, **15+ video reviews** that walk you step by step through each topic, and **5 downloadable resources** to help you apply the strategies.

Online Study Secrets Course

Course Features:

- Techniques to Conquer Procrastination
- Steps to Building a Study Plan
- 7 Effective Note-Taking Methods
- Test-Taking Tips
- Memory Techniques and Mnemonics
- 50 Quick and Unusual Study Tips
- How to Create SMART Goals
- How to Study Math
- And much more!

Everyone learns differently, so we've tailored our Study Secrets Course to ensure that every learner has what they need to prepare for their upcoming exam or semester.

To purchase this course and start studying, visit us at mometrix.com/university/studysecrets or simply scan this QR code with your smartphone.

If you have any questions or concerns, please contact us at support@mometrix.com.

M⊘metrix
TEST PREPARATION

ACCESS YOUR ONLINE RESOURCES

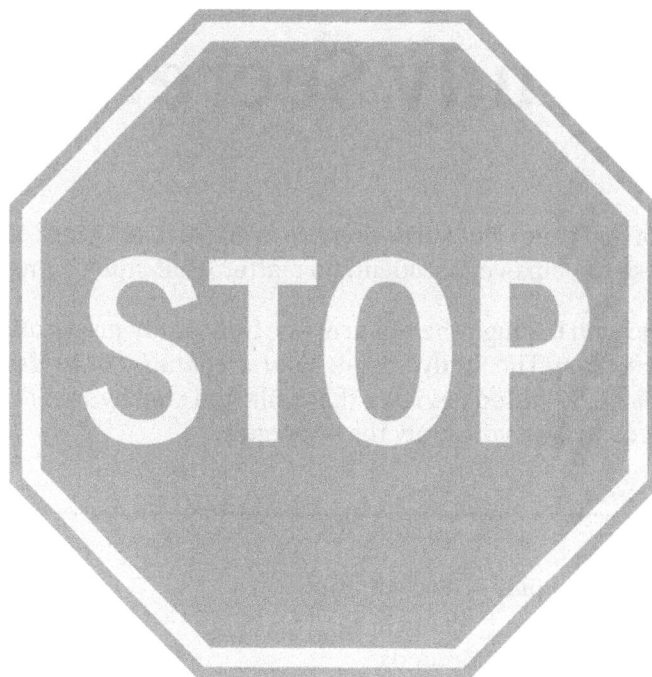

DON'T MISS OUT ON THE ONLINE RESOURCES INCLUDED WITH YOUR PURCHASE!

Your purchase of this product unlocks access to our Online Resources page. Elevate your study experience with our **interactive practice test interface**, along with all of the additional resources that we couldn't include in this book.

Flip to the Online Resources section at the end of this book to find the link and a QR code to get started!

Mometrix
TEST PREPARATION

Mometrix
TEST PREPARATION

NHA EKG

Study Guide 2025–2026

3 Full-Length Practice Tests

EKG Technician Exam Prep Secrets for the CET

Detailed Answer Explanations

Written and edited by Matthew Bowling

Printed in the United States of America

This paper meets the requirements of ANSI/NISO Z39.48-1992 (Permanence of Paper).

Mometrix offers volume discount pricing to institutions. For more information or a price quote, please contact our sales department at sales@mometrix.com or 888-248-1219.

Mometrix Media LLC is not affiliated with or endorsed by any official testing organization. All organizational and test names are trademarks of their respective owners.

Paperback
ISBN 13: 978-1-5167-2871-8
ISBN 10: 1-5167-2871-8

DEAR FUTURE EXAM SUCCESS STORY

First of all, **THANK YOU** for purchasing Mometrix study materials!

Second, congratulations! You are one of the few determined test-takers who are committed to doing whatever it takes to excel on your exam. **You have come to the right place.** We developed these study materials with one goal in mind: to deliver you the information you need in a format that's concise and easy to use.

In addition to optimizing your guide for the content of the test, we've outlined our recommended steps for breaking down the preparation process into small, attainable goals so you can make sure you stay on track.

We've also analyzed the entire test-taking process, identifying the most common pitfalls and showing how you can overcome them and be ready for any curveball the test throws you.

Standardized testing is one of the biggest obstacles on your road to success, which only increases the importance of doing well in the high-pressure, high-stakes environment of test day. Your results on this test could have a significant impact on your future, and this guide provides the information and practical advice to help you achieve your full potential on test day.

Your success is our success

We would love to hear from you! If you would like to share the story of your exam success or if you have any questions or comments in regard to our products, please contact us at **800-673-8175** or **support@mometrix.com**.

Thanks again for your business and we wish you continued success!

Sincerely,
The Mometrix Test Preparation Team

TABLE OF CONTENTS

Introduction

Thank you for purchasing this resource! You have made the choice to prepare yourself for a test that could have a huge impact on your future, and this guide is designed to help you be fully ready for test day. Obviously, it's important to have a solid understanding of the test material, but you also need to be prepared for the unique environment and stressors of the test, so that you can perform to the best of your abilities.

For this purpose, the first section that appears in this guide is the **Secret Keys**. We've devoted countless hours to meticulously researching what works and what doesn't, and we've boiled down our findings to the five most impactful steps you can take to improve your performance on the test. We start at the beginning with study planning and move through the preparation process, all the way to the testing strategies that will help you get the most out of what you know when you're finally sitting in front of the test.

We recommend that you start preparing for your test as far in advance as possible. However, if you've bought this guide as a last-minute study resource and only have a few days before your test, we recommend that you skip over the first two Secret Keys since they address a long-term study plan.

If you struggle with **test anxiety**, we strongly encourage you to check out our recommendations for how you can overcome it. Test anxiety is a formidable foe, but it can be beaten, and we want to make sure you have the tools you need to defeat it.

1

Secret Key #1 – Plan Big, Study Small

There's a lot riding on your performance. If you want to ace this test, you're going to need to keep your skills sharp and the material fresh in your mind. You need a plan that lets you review everything you need to know while still fitting in your schedule. We'll break this strategy down into three categories.

Information Organization

Start with the information you already have: the official test outline. From this, you can make a complete list of all the concepts you need to cover before the test. Organize these concepts into groups that can be studied together, and create a list of any related vocabulary you need to learn so you can brush up on any difficult terms. You'll want to keep this vocabulary list handy once you actually start studying since you may need to add to it along the way.

Time Management

Once you have your set of study concepts, decide how to spread them out over the time you have left before the test. Break your study plan into small, clear goals so you have a manageable task for each day and know exactly what you're doing. Then just focus on one small step at a time. When you manage your time this way, you don't need to spend hours at a time studying. Studying a small block of content for a short period each day helps you retain information better and avoid stressing over how much you have left to do. You can relax knowing that you have a plan to cover everything in time. In order for this strategy to be effective though, you have to start studying early and stick to your schedule. Avoid the exhaustion and futility that comes from last-minute cramming!

Study Environment

The environment you study in has a big impact on your learning. Studying in a coffee shop, while probably more enjoyable, is not likely to be as fruitful as studying in a quiet room. It's important to keep distractions to a minimum. You're only planning to study for a short block of time, so make the most of it. Don't pause to check your phone or get up to find a snack. It's also important to **avoid multitasking**. Research has consistently shown that multitasking will make your studying dramatically less effective. Your study area should also be comfortable and well-lit so you don't have the distraction of straining your eyes or sitting on an uncomfortable chair.

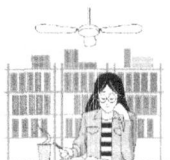

The time of day you study is also important. You want to be rested and alert. Don't wait until just before bedtime. Study when you'll be most likely to comprehend and remember. Even better, if you know what time of day your test will be, set that time aside for study. That way your brain will be used to working on that subject at that specific time and you'll have a better chance of recalling information.

Finally, it can be helpful to team up with others who are studying for the same test. Your actual studying should be done in as isolated an environment as possible, but the work of organizing the information and setting up the study plan can be divided up. In between study sessions, you can discuss with your teammates the concepts that you're all studying and quiz each other on the details. Just be sure that your teammates are as serious about the test as you are. If you find that your study time is being replaced with social time, you might need to find a new team.

Secret Key #2 – Make Your Studying Count

You're devoting a lot of time and effort to preparing for this test, so you want to be absolutely certain it will pay off. This means doing more than just reading the content and hoping you can remember it on test day. It's important to make every minute of study count. There are two main areas you can focus on to make your studying count.

Retention

It doesn't matter how much time you study if you can't remember the material. You need to make sure you are retaining the concepts. To check your retention of the information you're learning, try recalling it at later times with minimal prompting. Try carrying around flashcards and glance at one or two from time to time or ask a friend who's also studying for the test to quiz you.

To enhance your retention, look for ways to put the information into practice so that you can apply it rather than simply recalling it. If you're using the information in practical ways, it will be much easier to remember. Similarly, it helps to solidify a concept in your mind if you're not only reading it to yourself but also explaining it to someone else. Ask a friend to let you teach them about a concept you're a little shaky on (or speak aloud to an imaginary audience if necessary). As you try to summarize, define, give examples, and answer your friend's questions, you'll understand the concepts better and they will stay with you longer. Finally, step back for a big picture view and ask yourself how each piece of information fits with the whole subject. When you link the different concepts together and see them working together as a whole, it's easier to remember the individual components.

Finally, practice showing your work on any multi-step problems, even if you're just studying. Writing out each step you take to solve a problem will help solidify the process in your mind, and you'll be more likely to remember it during the test.

Modality

Modality simply refers to the means or method by which you study. Choosing a study modality that fits your own individual learning style is crucial. No two people learn best in exactly the same way, so it's important to know your strengths and use them to your advantage.

For example, if you learn best by visualization, focus on visualizing a concept in your mind and draw an image or a diagram. Try color-coding your notes, illustrating them, or creating symbols that will trigger your mind to recall a learned concept. If you learn best by hearing or discussing information, find a study partner who learns the same way or read aloud to yourself. Think about how to put the information in your own words. Imagine that you are giving a lecture on the topic and record yourself so you can listen to it later.

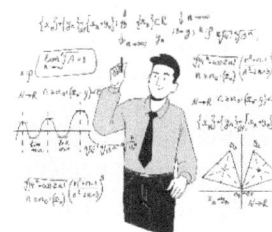

For any learning style, flashcards can be helpful. Organize the information so you can take advantage of spare moments to review. Underline key words or phrases. Use different colors for different categories. Mnemonic devices (such as creating a short list in which every item starts with the same letter) can also help with retention. Find what works best for you and use it to store the information in your mind most effectively and easily.

3

Secret Key #3 – Practice the Right Way

Your success on test day depends not only on how many hours you put into preparing, but also on whether you prepared the right way. It's good to check along the way to see if your studying is paying off. One of the most effective ways to do this is by taking practice tests to evaluate your progress. Practice tests are useful because they show exactly where you need to improve. Every time you take a practice test, pay special attention to these three groups of questions:

- The questions you got wrong
- The questions you had to guess on, even if you guessed right
- The questions you found difficult or slow to work through

This will show you exactly what your weak areas are, and where you need to devote more study time. Ask yourself why each of these questions gave you trouble. Was it because you didn't understand the material? Was it because you didn't remember the vocabulary? Do you need more repetitions on this type of question to build speed and confidence? Dig into those questions and figure out how you can strengthen your weak areas as you go back to review the material.

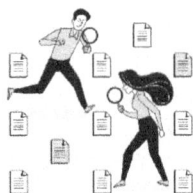

Additionally, many practice tests have a section explaining the answer choices. It can be tempting to read the explanation and think that you now have a good understanding of the concept. However, an explanation likely only covers part of the question's broader context. Even if the explanation makes perfect sense, **go back and investigate** every concept related to the question until you're positive you have a thorough understanding.

As you go along, keep in mind that the practice test is just that: practice. Memorizing these questions and answers will not be very helpful on the actual test because it is unlikely to have any of the same exact questions. If you only know the right answers to the sample questions, you won't be prepared for the real thing. **Study the concepts** until you understand them fully, and then you'll be able to answer any question that shows up on the test.

It's important to wait on the practice tests until you're ready. If you take a test on your first day of study, you may be overwhelmed by the amount of material covered and how much you need to learn. Work up to it gradually.

On test day, you'll need to be prepared for answering questions, managing your time, and using the test-taking strategies you've learned. It's a lot to balance, like a mental marathon that will have a big impact on your future. Like training for a marathon, you'll need to start slowly and work your way up. When test day arrives, you'll be ready.

Start with the strategies you've read in the first two Secret Keys—plan your course and study in the way that works best for you. If you have time, consider using multiple study resources to get different approaches to the same concepts. It can be helpful to see difficult concepts from more than one angle. Then find a good source for practice tests. Many times, the test website will suggest potential study resources or provide sample tests.

Practice Test Strategy

If you're able to find at least three practice tests, we recommend this strategy:

UNTIMED AND OPEN-BOOK PRACTICE

Take the first test with no time constraints and with your notes and study guide handy. Take your time and focus on applying the strategies you've learned.

TIMED AND OPEN-BOOK PRACTICE

Take the second practice test open-book as well, but set a timer and practice pacing yourself to finish in time.

TIMED AND CLOSED-BOOK PRACTICE

Take any other practice tests as if it were test day. Set a timer and put away your study materials. Sit at a table or desk in a quiet room, imagine yourself at the testing center, and answer questions as quickly and accurately as possible.

Keep repeating timed and closed-book tests on a regular basis until you run out of practice tests or it's time for the actual test. Your mind will be ready for the schedule and stress of test day, and you'll be able to focus on recalling the material you've learned.

5

Secret Key #4 – Pace Yourself

Once you're fully prepared for the material on the test, your biggest challenge on test day will be managing your time. Just knowing that the clock is ticking can make you panic even if you have plenty of time left. Work on pacing yourself so you can build confidence against the time constraints of the exam. Pacing is a difficult skill to master, especially in a high-pressure environment, so **practice is vital**.

Set time expectations for your pace based on how much time is available. For example, if a section has 60 questions and the time limit is 30 minutes, you know you have to average 30 seconds or less per question in order to answer them all. Although 30 seconds is the hard limit, set 25 seconds per question as your goal, so you reserve extra time to spend on harder questions. When you budget extra time for the harder questions, you no longer have any reason to stress when those questions take longer to answer.

Don't let this time expectation distract you from working through the test at a calm, steady pace, but keep it in mind so you don't spend too much time on any one question. Recognize that taking extra time on one question you don't understand may keep you from answering two that you do understand later in the test. If your time limit for a question is up and you're still not sure of the answer, mark it and move on, and come back to it later if the time and the test format allow. If the testing format doesn't allow you to return to earlier questions, just make an educated guess; then put it out of your mind and move on.

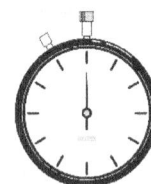

On the easier questions, be careful not to rush. It may seem wise to hurry through them so you have more time for the challenging ones, but it's not worth missing one if you know the concept and just didn't take the time to read the question fully. Work efficiently but make sure you understand the question and have looked at all of the answer choices, since more than one may seem right at first.

Even if you're paying attention to the time, you may find yourself a little behind at some point. You should speed up to get back on track, but do so wisely. Don't panic; just take a few seconds less on each question until you're caught up. Don't guess without thinking, but do look through the answer choices and eliminate any you know are wrong. If you can get down to two choices, it is often worthwhile to guess from those. Once you've chosen an answer, move on and don't dwell on any that you skipped or had to hurry through. If a question was taking too long, chances are it was one of the harder ones, so you weren't as likely to get it right anyway.

On the other hand, if you find yourself getting ahead of schedule, it may be beneficial to slow down a little. The more quickly you work, the more likely you are to make a careless mistake that will affect your score. You've budgeted time for each question, so don't be afraid to spend that time. Practice an efficient but careful pace to get the most out of the time you have.

Secret Key #5 – Have a Plan for Guessing

When you're taking the test, you may find yourself stuck on a question. Some of the answer choices seem better than others, but you don't see the one answer choice that is obviously correct. What do you do?

The scenario described above is very common, yet most test takers have not effectively prepared for it. Developing and practicing a plan for guessing may be one of the single most effective uses of your time as you get ready for the exam.

In developing your plan for guessing, there are three questions to address:

- When should you start the guessing process?
- How should you narrow down the choices?
- Which answer should you choose?

When to Start the Guessing Process

Unless your plan for guessing is to select C every time (which, despite its merits, is not what we recommend), you need to leave yourself enough time to apply your answer elimination strategies. Since you have a limited amount of time for each question, that means that if you're going to give yourself the best shot at guessing correctly, you have to decide quickly whether or not you will guess.

Of course, the best-case scenario is that you don't have to guess at all, so first, see if you can answer the question based on your knowledge of the subject and basic reasoning skills. Focus on the key words in the question and try to jog your memory of related topics. Give yourself a chance to bring the knowledge to mind, but once you realize that you don't have (or you can't access) the knowledge you need to answer the question, it's time to start the guessing process.

It's almost always better to start the guessing process too early than too late. It only takes a few seconds to remember something and answer the question from knowledge. Carefully eliminating wrong answer choices takes longer. Plus, going through the process of eliminating answer choices can actually help jog your memory.

Summary: Start the guessing process as soon as you decide that you can't answer the question based on your knowledge.

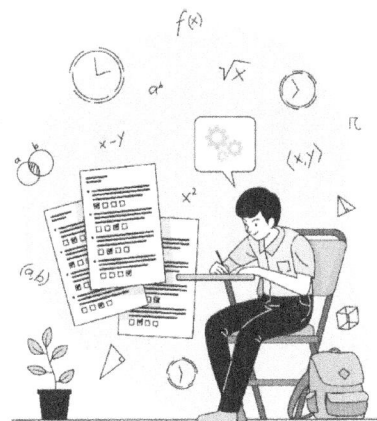

7

How to Narrow Down the Choices

The next chapter in this book (**Test-Taking Strategies**) includes a wide range of strategies for how to approach questions and how to look for answer choices to eliminate. You will definitely want to read those carefully, practice them, and figure out which ones work best for you. Here though, we're going to address a mindset rather than a particular strategy.

Your odds of guessing an answer correctly depend on how many options you are choosing from.

Number of options left	5	4	3	2	1
Odds of guessing correctly	20%	25%	33%	50%	100%

You can see from this chart just how valuable it is to be able to eliminate incorrect answers and make an educated guess, but there are two things that many test takers do that cause them to miss out on the benefits of guessing:

- Accidentally eliminating the correct answer
- Selecting an answer based on an impression

We'll look at the first one here, and the second one in the next section.

To avoid accidentally eliminating the correct answer, we recommend a thought exercise called **the $5 challenge**. In this challenge, you only eliminate an answer choice from contention if you are willing to bet $5 on it being wrong. Why $5? Five dollars is a small but not insignificant amount of money. It's an amount you could afford to lose but wouldn't want to throw away. And while losing $5 once might not hurt too much, doing it twenty times will set you back $100. In the same way, each small decision you make—eliminating a choice here, guessing on a question there—won't by itself impact your score very much, but when you put them all together, they can make a big difference. By holding each answer choice elimination decision to a higher standard, you can reduce the risk of accidentally eliminating the correct answer.

The $5 challenge can also be applied in a positive sense: If you are willing to bet $5 that an answer choice *is* correct, go ahead and mark it as correct.

Summary: Only eliminate an answer choice if you are willing to bet $5 that it is wrong.

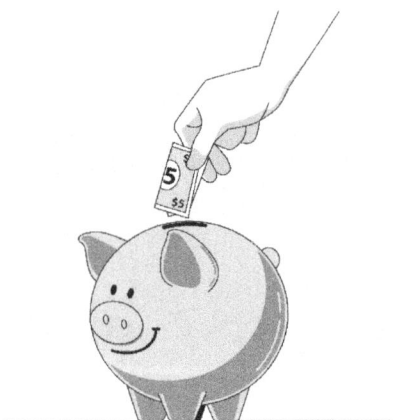

Which Answer to Choose

You're taking the test. You've run into a hard question and decided you'll have to guess. You've eliminated all the answer choices you're willing to bet $5 on. Now you have to pick an answer. Why do we even need to talk about this? Why can't you just pick whichever one you feel like when the time comes?

The answer to these questions is that if you don't come into the test with a plan, you'll rely on your impression to select an answer choice, and if you do that, you risk falling into a trap. The test writers know that everyone who takes their test will be guessing on some of the questions, so they intentionally write wrong answer choices to seem plausible. You still have to pick an answer though, and if the wrong answer choices are designed to look right, how can you ever be sure that you're not falling for their trap? The best solution we've found to this dilemma is to take the decision out of your hands entirely. Here is the process we recommend:

Once you've eliminated any choices that you are confident (willing to bet $5) are wrong, select the first remaining choice as your answer.

Whether you choose to select the first remaining choice, the second, or the last, the important thing is that you use some preselected standard. Using this approach guarantees that you will not be enticed into selecting an answer choice that looks right, because you are not basing your decision on how the answer choices look.

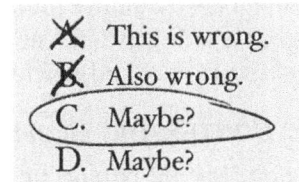

~~A.~~ This is wrong.
~~B.~~ Also wrong.
C. Maybe?
D. Maybe?

This is not meant to make you question your knowledge. Instead, it is to help you recognize the difference between your knowledge and your impressions. There's a huge difference between thinking an answer is right because of what you know, and thinking an answer is right because it looks or sounds like it should be right.

Summary: To ensure that your selection is appropriately random, make a predetermined selection from among all answer choices you have not eliminated.

Test-Taking Strategies

This section contains a list of test-taking strategies that you may find helpful as you work through the test. By taking what you know and applying logical thought, you can maximize your chances of answering any question correctly!

It is very important to realize that every question is different and every person is different: no single strategy will work on every question, and no single strategy will work for every person. That's why we've included all of them here, so you can try them out and determine which ones work best for different types of questions and which ones work best for you.

Question Strategies

⊘ READ CAREFULLY

Read the question and the answer choices carefully. Don't miss the question because you misread the terms. You have plenty of time to read each question thoroughly and make sure you understand what is being asked. Yet a happy medium must be attained, so don't waste too much time. You must read carefully and efficiently.

⊘ CONTEXTUAL CLUES

Look for contextual clues. If the question includes a word you are not familiar with, look at the immediate context for some indication of what the word might mean. Contextual clues can often give you all the information you need to decipher the meaning of an unfamiliar word. Even if you can't determine the meaning, you may be able to narrow down the possibilities enough to make a solid guess at the answer to the question.

⊘ PREFIXES

If you're having trouble with a word in the question or answer choices, try dissecting it. Take advantage of every clue that the word might include. Prefixes can be a huge help. Usually, they allow you to determine a basic meaning. *Pre-* means before, *post-* means after, *pro-* is positive, *de-* is negative. From prefixes, you can get an idea of the general meaning of the word and try to put it into context.

⊘ HEDGE WORDS

Watch out for critical hedge words, such as *likely, may, can, sometimes, often, almost, mostly, usually, generally, rarely,* and *sometimes*. Question writers insert these hedge phrases to cover every possibility. Often an answer choice will be wrong simply because it leaves no room for exception. Be on guard for answer choices that have definitive words such as *exactly* and *always*.

⊘ SWITCHBACK WORDS

Stay alert for *switchbacks*. These are the words and phrases frequently used to alert you to shifts in thought. The most common switchback words are *but, although,* and *however*. Others include *nevertheless, on the other hand, even though, while, in spite of, despite,* and *regardless of*. Switchback words are important to catch because they can change the direction of the question or an answer choice.

⊘ FACE VALUE

When in doubt, use common sense. Accept the situation in the problem at face value. Don't read too much into it. These problems will not require you to make wild assumptions. If you have to go beyond creativity and warp time or space in order to have an answer choice fit the question, then you should move on and consider the other answer choices. These are normal problems rooted in reality. The applicable relationship or explanation may not be readily apparent, but it is there for you to figure out. Use your common sense to interpret anything that isn't clear.

Answer Choice Strategies

⊘ ANSWER SELECTION

The most thorough way to pick an answer choice is to identify and eliminate wrong answers until only one is left, then confirm it is the correct answer. Sometimes an answer choice may immediately seem right, but be careful. The test writers will usually put more than one reasonable answer choice on each question, so take a second to read all of them and make sure that the other choices are not equally obvious. As long as you have time left, it is better to read every answer choice than to pick the first one that looks right without checking the others.

⊘ ANSWER CHOICE FAMILIES

An answer choice family consists of two (in rare cases, three) answer choices that are very similar in construction and cannot all be true at the same time. If you see two answer choices that are direct opposites or parallels, one of them is usually the correct answer. For instance, if one answer choice says that quantity x increases and another either says that quantity x decreases (opposite) or says that quantity y increases (parallel), then those answer choices would fall into the same family. An answer choice that doesn't match the construction of the answer choice family is more likely to be incorrect. Most questions will not have answer choice families, but when they do appear, you should be prepared to recognize them.

⊘ ELIMINATE ANSWERS

Eliminate answer choices as soon as you realize they are wrong, but make sure you consider all possibilities. If you are eliminating answer choices and realize that the last one you are left with is also wrong, don't panic. Start over and consider each choice again. There may be something you missed the first time that you will realize on the second pass.

⊘ AVOID FACT TRAPS

Don't be distracted by an answer choice that is factually true but doesn't answer the question. You are looking for the choice that answers the question. Stay focused on what the question is asking for so you don't accidentally pick an answer that is true but incorrect. Always go back to the question and make sure the answer choice you've selected actually answers the question and is not merely a true statement.

⊘ EXTREME STATEMENTS

In general, you should avoid answers that put forth extreme actions as standard practice or proclaim controversial ideas as established fact. An answer choice that states the "process should be used in certain situations, if…" is much more likely to be correct than one that states the "process should be discontinued completely." The first is a calm rational statement and doesn't even make a definitive, uncompromising stance, using a hedge word *if* to provide wiggle room, whereas the second choice is far more extreme.

⊘ BENCHMARK

As you read through the answer choices and you come across one that seems to answer the question well, mentally select that answer choice. This is not your final answer, but it's the one that will help you evaluate the other answer choices. The one that you selected is your benchmark or standard for judging each of the other answer choices. Every other answer choice must be compared to your benchmark. That choice is correct until proven otherwise by another answer choice beating it. If you find a better answer, then that one becomes your new benchmark. Once you've decided that no other choice answers the question as well as your benchmark, you have your final answer.

⊘ PREDICT THE ANSWER

Before you even start looking at the answer choices, it is often best to try to predict the answer. When you come up with the answer on your own, it is easier to avoid distractions and traps because you will know exactly what to look for. The right answer choice is unlikely to be word-for-word what you came up with, but it should be a close match. Even if you are confident that you have the right answer, you should still take the time to read each option before moving on.

General Strategies

⊘ TOUGH QUESTIONS

If you are stumped on a problem or it appears too hard or too difficult, don't waste time. Move on! Remember though, if you can quickly check for obviously incorrect answer choices, your chances of guessing correctly are greatly improved. Before you completely give up, at least try to knock out a couple of possible answers. Eliminate what you can and then guess at the remaining answer choices before moving on.

⊘ CHECK YOUR WORK

Since you will probably not know every term listed and the answer to every question, it is important that you get credit for the ones that you do know. Don't miss any questions through careless mistakes. If at all possible, try to take a second to look back over your answer selection and make sure you've selected the correct answer choice and haven't made a costly careless mistake (such as marking an answer choice that you didn't mean to mark). This quick double check should more than pay for itself in caught mistakes for the time it costs.

⊘ PACE YOURSELF

It's easy to be overwhelmed when you're looking at a page full of questions; your mind is confused and full of random thoughts, and the clock is ticking down faster than you would like. Calm down and maintain the pace that you have set for yourself. Especially as you get down to the last few minutes of the test, don't let the small numbers on the clock make you panic. As long as you are on track by monitoring your pace, you are guaranteed to have time for each question.

⊘ DON'T RUSH

It is very easy to make errors when you are in a hurry. Maintaining a fast pace in answering questions is pointless if it makes you miss questions that you would have gotten right otherwise. Test writers like to include distracting information and wrong answers that seem right. Taking a little extra time to avoid careless mistakes can make all the difference in your test score. Find a pace that allows you to be confident in the answers that you select.

⊘ KEEP MOVING

Panicking will not help you pass the test, so do your best to stay calm and keep moving. Taking deep breaths and going through the answer elimination steps you practiced can help to break through a stress barrier and keep your pace.

Final Notes

The combination of a solid foundation of content knowledge and the confidence that comes from practicing your plan for applying that knowledge is the key to maximizing your performance on test day. As your foundation of content knowledge is built up and strengthened, you'll find that the strategies included in this chapter become more and more effective in helping you quickly sift through the distractions and traps of the test to isolate the correct answer.

Now that you're preparing to move forward into the test content chapters of this book, be sure to keep your goal in mind. As you read, think about how you will be able to apply this information on the test. If you've already seen sample questions for the test and you have an idea of the question format and style, try to come up with questions of your own that you can answer based on what you're reading. This will give you valuable practice applying your knowledge in the same ways you can expect to on test day.

Good luck and good studying!

Safety, Compliance, and Coordinated Patient Care

Adhere to HIPAA Regulations and Infection Control

HIPAA

HIPAA stands for **Health Insurance Portability and Accountability Act** of 1996. HIPAA's Title I regulates healthcare accessibility, especially in the cases of job change and loss; Title II regulates patient privacy rights. HIPAA requires the following:

- Every patient's medical record must bear a unique identifier to prevent misidentification
- Patients must be given access to their protected health information (medical records) at any time, upon request
- Only relevant health information can be disclosed to authorized parties
- A record must be kept of every disclosure
- Every patient or the parents/guardian must receive a *Notice of Privacy Practices*, outlining how the protected health information will be used
- Physical access to protected health information must be limited (including electronic files via password protection or swipe cards, firewall, and SSL encryption)
- Retired electronic equipment must have all data records wiped clean

> **Review Video: HIPAA**
> Visit mometrix.com/academy and enter code: 412009

OSHA

The US Department of Labor's **Occupational Safety and Health Administration (OSHA)** sets standards for:

- Proper hand washing
- Wearing gloves and other personal protective equipment (PPE)
- Bagging specimens in biohazard bags
- Disposing of needles and lancets in a sharps container
- Cleaning up spills to prevent spread of bloodborne pathogens
- Harmful chemical control
- Safe equipment use
- Adequate work space

Check for updates regularly at OSHA's website. These updates are required to be adopted as part of the facility's standards of practice.

15

MODES OF INFECTION TRANSMISSION

Modes of infection transmission include the following (with possible infectious diseases in parenthesis):

- **Direct contact**: Direct touching, kissing (mononucleosis) and sexual intercourse (gonorrhea, syphilis, chlamydia, HIV). Vertical transmission involves mother to infant during pregnancy, delivery, or breastfeeding (HIV, hepatitis B, gonorrhea, herpes).
- **Indirect contact**: A contaminated fomite (inanimate object), such as a doorknob, syringe, or catheter, spreads infection (*Clostridioides difficile*).
- **Airborne**: Particles less than 5 µm in size inhaled from cough, sneeze, or exhalation. Particles stay suspended in the air and travel large distances (tuberculosis, measles, COVID-19).
- **Droplet**: Particles greater than 5 µm in size are inhaled from a cough, sneeze, or exhalation (influenza, mumps, meningitis, pertussis, pneumonia, rubella). Droplets travel less than 3 feet and do not stay suspended, therefore are less contagious than airborne particles.
- **Vehicle**: Contact with contaminated water, air, or food (*E. coli* diarrhea, Cryptosporidiosis, hepatitis A).
- **Vector (mechanical)**: Contact with an animal, insect, or device that carries infection from one host to another (such as a fly carrying bacteria from feces of an infected host to food [dysentery]).
- **Vector (biological)**: Infected biological vector (such as a tick or flea) transmits infection directly to another host (Chagas disease, malaria, West Nile virus, Lyme disease).

CHAIN OF INFECTION AND NATURAL BARRIERS TO INFECTION

There are six components to the chain of infection:

- **Infectious microorganisms**: Bacteria, viruses, fungi, parasites
- **Reservoir**: The place the microorganism lives and reproduces (water, feces, body fluids, toilet seats, door knobs, blood)
- **Portal of exit**: The place where the microorganism leaves the reservoir (nose, mouth, rectum, blood, sputum)
- **Transmission mode**: The method (direct or indirect) by which a microorganism travels from one host to another
- **Portal of entry**: The site at which a microorganism enters a host (wounds, mucous membranes, feeding tubes, urinary catheter, ventilation tube, IV)
- **Susceptible host**: The host at risk of developing the infection

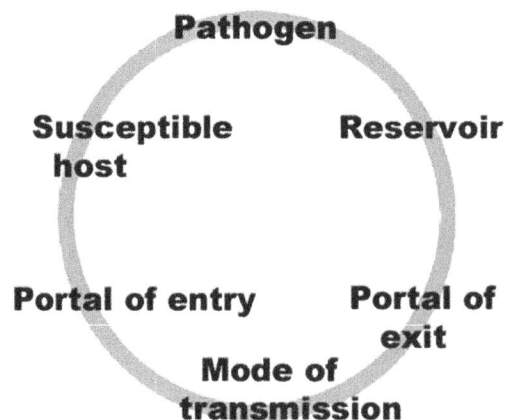

Natural barriers to infection include an effective immune system, intact skin, adequate cough reflex and air filtering (nose and lungs), digestive acids and enzymes (destroy some pathogens), healthy mucous membranes (prevent infections), blood components (white blood cells), inflammation response (walls off infection), urethra (provides protection of urinary system), and fever (increases body defense system).

INFECTION CONTROL PRECAUTIONS

Various levels of infection control precautions exist to aid in the prevention of the spread of infection amongst health care workers and facilities:

- **Standard or universal precautions** are means through which healthcare workers control the spread of disease by assuming every patient's samples are infectious, and following the OSHA standards for proper hand washing, wearing gloves and other personal protective equipment (PPE), bagging specimens in biohazard bags, and disposing of needles and lancets in a sharps container.
- **Contact precautions** prevent direct and indirect contact transmission of infectious pathogens such as those found with herpes simplex, infected wounds, and infectious diarrhea. PPE includes wearing gloves and gown upon room entry and properly discarding before exiting the patient room.
- **Droplet precautions** are used to prevent the transmission of pathogens transmitted by respiratory droplets from coughing, sneezing, or talking. PPE includes a mask for the patient when being transported outside patient room, and a mask for medical personnel when entering the patient room.
- **Airborne precautions** are used for airborne transmission microbes such as tuberculosis, which require a negative pressure private room and a HEPA or fit-tested N95 mask.

Isolating infectious patients is essential to reduce the risk of infection.

- **Strict isolation** segregates infectious patients to one room, and visitors are restricted.
- **Modified isolation** attempts to limit infection with protective techniques, like donning gloves, gowns, and masks when handling the patient's body fluids.
- **Reverse isolation** protects a patient from others in a clean room, as after kidney transplant.

MEDICAL ASEPSIS

Medical asepsis is defined as the absence of disease-causing microorganisms and is often referred to as **clean**. Medical asepsis is used to prevent the spread of hospital-acquired (nosocomial) disease and cross-infections (different pathogens passed between two patients):

- Wash hands using proper hand hygiene whenever visibly soiled, before and after any contact with patients, and after gloves are removed.
- Disinfect patient care materials before use with the proper chemical agent, according to the manufacturer's specifications.
- Maintain a clean patient care environment, with adequate space, ventilation, sunlight, and cool temperature.
- Dispose of infectious material as soon as soiling is discovered in the proper bin (concurrent cleaning).
- Disinfect patient care materials after a patient leaves the office, dies, or is transferred to another floor or facility (terminal cleaning).
- Use clean and dirty utility rooms to separate unused equipment from used equipment and prevent contamination.
- Store clean linen separate from used linen, and limit access to the clean linen room to authorized personnel only.

HAND HYGIENE

Practicing appropriate hand hygiene is the most effective way to prevent the spread of infection when done properly. Prior to donning gloves and approaching a patient for ECG collection, the ECG tech must practice appropriate hand hygiene, usually in the form of applying a 60% alcohol-based hand sanitizer. Rub gel over all the surfaces of hands and fingers until hands are dry, about 20 seconds, and then don gloves. Of note, although hand sanitizers are effective against most pathogenic microorganisms, they are not effective against *Clostridioides difficile*. Upon leaving a patient's room, the gloves must be discarded and hand sanitizer applied, unless the ECG technician came in contact with bodily fluids or the patient was on contact precautions that require hand washing. In these cases, the ECG technician must wash hands, as hand sanitizer is not sufficient.

To **wash hands correctly**, wet the hands with clean running water and apply soap. Lather hands by rubbing them together with soap, scrubbing the backs of hands, between fingers, and under nails for at least 20 seconds. Note any cuts, rashes, broken or long nails that need treatment before resuming work. Rinse well under clean running water and dry hands with paper towels, not a blow dryer. Use a clean paper towel to turn off the taps and to open the exit door.

Hand hygiene should be performed before and after each client contact, anytime they are visibly soiled, and before and after donning and removing gloves. To avoid contamination when removing gloves, remove them by turning them inside out from the wrists.

Scope of Practice and Ethical Standards

NHA SCOPE OF PRACTICE FOR THE CERTIFIED ECG TECHNICIAN

The NHA scope of practice for the certified ECG technician includes:

- **Administer ECGs**: Prepare patients, set up equipment, carry out testing
- **Conduct stress tests**: Prepare patients, explain procedures, apply electrodes, monitor heart performance
- **Prepare patients for ambulatory monitoring, such as with the Holter monitor**: Prepare patients and instruct on the use and care of the provided monitoring equipment
- **Equipment maintenance**: Check machine settings and calibration; ensure upkeep of all ECG equipment
- **Patient safety**: Adhere to all infection control protocols
- **Communication**: Use therapeutic communication and active listening to prepare patients, address their concerns, and ensure their understanding; collect information to assist other healthcare professionals with patient care
- **Interpretation**: Recognizing normal and abnormal heart rhythms and alerting health professionals as needed
- **Documentation**: Record the results of tests in patient health records
- **Education**: Provide clear and complete education regarding procedures to patients to ensure their comfort and safety
- **Emergency response**: Recognize indications of cardiopulmonary compromise and initiate basic life support (cardiopulmonary resuscitation) if indicated

NHA CODE OF ETHICS

The NHA Code of Ethics for certified professionals applies to all NHA certifications except for the pharmacy technician; it is intended to protect the profession and the public. The NHA Code of Ethics includes:

- Working toward the betterment of society, the profession, and members of the profession
- Upholding professional standards and veracity in all professional interactions
- Learning continually to stay up to date with knowledge, advance science, improve one's skills, and understand practical applications
- Participating in activities and contributing toward personal health, society, and the allied health industry
- Always acting in the best interests of the general public
- Respecting and protecting the dignity, privacy, and safety of all patients

Failure to adhere to the NHA Code of Ethics may be considered misconduct and may result in disciplinary action against the individual. Disciplinary actions may vary but can include certification revocation.

CORE ETHICAL PRINCIPLES

Core ethical principles include:

- **Beneficence**: Performing actions that are for the purpose of benefitting another person. In the care of a patient, any procedure or treatment should be done with the ultimate goal of benefitting the patient.
- **Nonmaleficence**: Providing care in a manner that does not cause direct intentional harm to the patient. Care must be intended only for good effect, and good effects must have more benefit than bad effects that result.
- **Autonomy**: The right of the individual to make decisions about his or her own care. In the case of children, the child cannot make autonomous decisions, so the parents serve as the legal decision maker.
- **Justice**: Relates to the distribution of the limited resources of healthcare benefits to the members of society. Resources must be distributed fairly and decisions made according to what is most just.
- **Privacy/confidentiality**: Protecting information (conversations, assessments) and body (close door, pull curtains, use drapes to avoid exposing patient) and protecting personal information about a patient and the patient's health condition.

PATIENTS' RIGHTS

The Advisory Commission on Consumer Protection and Quality on Health Care Industry outlined eight **rights and responsibilities of American patients** as follows:

- The right to information
- The right to choose
- The right to access emergency services
- The right to fully participate in decisions regarding one's own health care
- The right to care without discrimination
- The right to privacy
- The right to speedy complaint resolution
- The responsibility for maintaining one's health to retain those rights

The American Hospital Association replaced its *Patients' Bill of Rights* in 2008 with a brochure called *The Patient Care Partnership*, which is available in many languages on the AHA website. Information about how HIPAA protects patients' rights can be found on the HHS website.

ADVANCE DIRECTIVE, CODE BLUE, AND DNR ORDER

An **advance directive** is a legal document in which the patient communicates to his or her family and physician what kind of medical intervention he or she desires. A **living will** is a type of advance directive that terminally ill patients often make. Specific laws regarding advance directives vary by state, but the patient must always be competent.

A **"do not resuscitate" order** is a type of advance directive. A DNR order must be written in the patient's chart by the attending physician in order to be valid. All discussions with the patient and the family should be clearly documented in the chart. In the absence of a written DNR order, call a full Code Blue and proceed with resuscitation.

Code blue is a distress call that indicates a patient is in cardiac arrest. Call the resuscitation team immediately. Some patient rooms have code blue buttons that can be pushed to activate the code blue. Additional codes exist for respiratory distress, patient/family violence, elopement, or the abduction of a newborn or child.

INFORMED CONSENT

Informed consent protects patients by ensuring that they or those legally responsible for them are fully educated about tests, treatments, and procedures. The patient has the legal right to know about his or her own condition. The exceptions are life-threatening emergencies and legal incompetence. Informed consent also protects healthcare professionals from lawsuits should a known risk/complication from the procedure occur.

Informed consent is obtained when the patient is given written and/or verbal information in regards to the treatment plan, risks, benefits, and alternative treatment options, the provider truthfully answers any questions, and the patient/parent/guardian comprehends the discussion. Most relevant to the ECG technician is that informed consent is required prior to a cardiac stress test. The patient or legal guardian must be informed of the purpose of the test, its benefits, and its possible risks, then voluntarily sign the consent form, without duress or coercion. Consent should be obtained by the provider performing the stress test, with a third party witness present. Always keep the original informed consent form in the patient's chart.

Communicate Appropriately with Patients and Members of the Health Care Team

COMMUNICATION CYCLE

The communication process, which includes the **sender-receiver feedback loop**, is based on Claude Shannon's information theory (1948) in which he described three necessary steps:

1. Encoding a message
2. Transmitting the message through a channel
3. Decoding the message

The resultant communication process begins with the sender, who serves as the encoder and determines the content of the message. The medium is the form the message takes (digital, written, audiovisual), and the channel is the method of delivery (mail, radio, TV, internet, phone). The recipient (receiver) who acts as the decoder determines the meaning from the message. Feedback helps to determine whether or not the communication is successful and the message understood as intended. This process is referred to as the send-receiver feedback loop. Context is the environment (physical and psychological) in which the communication occurs, and interference is any factor that impacts the communication process. Interference may be external (such as environmental noise) or internal (such as emotional distress or anxiety).

THERAPEUTIC COMMUNICATION
COMMUNICATION TECHNIQUES IN THERAPEUTIC RELATIONSHIPS

The following are appropriate communication techniques to encourage therapeutic relationships:

- **Use active listening**: Paraphrase and repeat back information transmitted by the patient. Ask for clarification when the message is confusing. Summarize what was agreed to at the end of the conversation.
- **Watch for nonverbal cues**: Nonverbal cues are gestures, grimaces, posturing, appearance, and eye movements that comprise 85% of all communication. Nonverbal cues can denote pain, fear, lying, depression, or subterfuge by a caregiver. Gently ask the patient to clarify when verbal and nonverbal cues do not match. Children and psychiatric patients may develop tic disorders (involuntary gestures and movements). If which movements are truly cues and which are tics cannot be deciphered, ask the doctor.
- **Ask open-ended questions**: Encourage the patient to explain their thoughts/feelings/understanding by asking open-ended questions rather than asking questions that require only a yes or no answer (close-ended questions).
- **Consider influences**: Put communication in the context of the patient's developmental age, emotions, values, ethics, health, education, culture, environment, social and familial status, and drug levels.

NON-THERAPEUTIC COMMUNICATION

The following are non-therapeutic communications techniques that must be avoided:

- **Ask leading questions**: Never shape the patient's answers to questions, or try to change the patient's interpretation of the situation by "putting words into the patient's mouth."
- **Demand an explanation**: Do not ask "why" questions in an accusing tone.
- **Give advice**: The physician advises and the ECG technician supports.
- **Demand an immediate response**: Allow the patient sufficient time for silent reflection before responding.
- **Disinterested body language**: Do not appear distracted or make the patient feel inconsequential with impatient motions, bored posture, or rolling eyes.
- **Minimize the patient's feelings**: Do not compare feelings and experiences.
- **Negatively empower**: Do not help the patient to manipulate another person.
- **Make false promises**: Never promise the patient that the doctor will definitely cure the condition, or make other promises that cannot be kept.
- **Play into stereotypes**: Racist, sexist, and religious prejudice must not influence the treatment of the patient.
- **Deliberately mislead**: Always disclose upcoming treatments, tests, or procedures.

EXAMPLES OF NON-THERAPEUTIC COMMUNICATION

Examples of non-therapeutic communication include the following:

- **Making negative judgments**: "You should stop arguing with the nurses."
- **Devaluing patient's feelings**: "Everyone gets upset at times."
- **Disagreeing directly**: "That can't be true," or "I think you are wrong."
- **Defending against criticism**: "The doctor is not being rude; he's just very busy today."
- **Subject-changing** to avoid dealing with uncomfortable topics:
  - Patient: "I'm never going to get well."
  - ECG technician: "Your parents will be here in just a few minutes."
- **Making inappropriate literal responses**, even as a joke, especially if the patient is at all confused or having difficulty expressing ideas:
  - Patient: "There are bugs crawling under my skin."
  - ECG technician: "I'll get some bug spray."
- **Challenging to establish reality**, which often just increases confusion and frustration: "If you were dying, you wouldn't be able to yell and kick!"

IMPORTANCE OF NONVERBAL COMMUNICATION

Any type of message transmitted between two people that does not involve words is considered **nonverbal communication**. As much as 85% of successful communication depends on nonverbal cues. Remember that the patient is likely apprehensive and English may not be his or her first language. The patient may have difficulty speaking due to injury, drugs, age, deformity, developmental disability, or the instruments used during a procedure. Watch the patient's facial expressions, gestures, posture, and position. Tight posture and/or crossed arms and legs suggest resistance. Conversely, relaxed posture and uncrossed appendages suggest openness. Additionally, one's own posture affects the patient. Sit closely beside the patient, rather than towering directly over him or her in an intimidating manner. Explain what is going to be done. A patient feels more comfortable when he or she is well informed beforehand. Maintain the proper social distancing (territoriality) between oneself and the patient during discussions (about 3 feet apart).

PROPER THERAPEUTIC RESPONSES WITH CERTAIN POPULATIONS

Therapeutic responses for specific populations include the following:

- **Pediatric/Adolescent**: Use vocabulary appropriate to age and encourage adolescents to make decisions whenever possible. Avoid approaching young children too abruptly and chat with the child and caregiver to ease the child's fear. Explain in advance any actions to be taken, such applying the leads of the ECG and letting the child know that this will not hurt, and allow the child to see and hold the equipment when possible.
- **Geriatric**: Treat patients with respect, address them by their names ("Mrs. Jones") and avoid terms like *honey* and *dear*. Be alert for barriers to communication, such as hearing deficits, and encourage patients to ask questions and discuss concerns. Avoid rushing and interrupting and utilize active listening skills.
- **Terminally ill**: Avoid being excessively sympathetic ("You poor thing"), but remain patient and empathetic. Utilize active listening and allow the patient time to express feelings or concerns. Understand that patients may be in pain, weak, frightened, nauseated, and/or depressed and may, for that reason, overreact or underreact.

SERVING MULTICULTURAL PATIENTS' NEEDS

When working in a diverse environment, the ECG technician must respect and tolerate **multicultural beliefs and values**, even if the patient is nonverbal. Most patients and their families willingly share their beliefs, so the ECG technician should not be embarrassed to ask about their preferences. Speak slowly while facing the patient, and do not address the translator first (if a translator is necessary). Order translations of patient guides and forms. Post pictorial direction signs. Allow multicultural families as much latitude as possible, without causing undue stress for other patients. If there is the possibility that a ritual will be noisy or alarming for other patients, respectfully guide the family to the Quiet Room. Realize some cultures have beliefs about specific food having healing or soothing qualities. Stay alert for symptoms of poisoning from traditional Chinese, Indian, Pacific Islander, and Mexican herbal medicines, which often contain mercury.

COMMUNICATING WITH INDIVIDUALS WITH DISABILITIES

The *Americans with Disabilities Act* of 1990 affects hiring, promotion, pay, and reasonable accommodations. It is enforced at business and service providers with more than 15 workers, on public transit, and with telecommunications.

The US Department of Labor suggests the following techniques when communicating with individuals with disabilities:

- Gain the person's attention before speaking by gently tapping the shoulder or arm.
- State clearly who you are. Speak in a normal tone of voice.
- Wait until one's offer of assistance is accepted. Then listen to or ask for instructions.
- Treat adults as adults. Address people who have disabilities by their first names only when extending the same familiarity to all others.
- Do not lead the person without first asking; allow the person to hold your arm and control her or his own movements.
- Be prepared to repeat what you say, orally or in writing.
- Use positive phrases, such as *person with a developmental disability*, rather than negative phrases, such as *mentally defective*.

COMMUNICATION TECHNIQUES FOR INDIVIDUALS WITH HEARING IMPAIRMENT

Hearing impaired patients may have some hearing and may use hearing aids while deaf patients typically have little or no hearing. Some patients are able to use lip reading to various degrees, so the ECG technician should always face the patient (at 3–6 feet) and speak slowly and clearly, using gestures (not excessively) to augment speech:

- **Hearing impaired**: Assistive devices (hearing aids, writing material) should be available and used during communication. Use a normal tone of voice and speak in short sentences. Minimize environmental noises.
- **Deaf**: If patients are deaf, sign language interpreters should be used for important communication (face the patient, not the interpreter). Assistive devices, such as writing materials, TDD phone/relay service, should be available for use. Always announce presence on entering a room by waving, clapping, tapping the foot (whatever works best for the patient). Ensure alarms have visual feedback (lights). Do not chew, smoke, or eat while speaking to the patient.

COMMUNICATION TECHNIQUES FOR INDIVIDUALS WITH VISION IMPAIRMENT

Visual impairment is unrelated to intelligence or hearing, so the ECG technician should speak with age-appropriate vocabulary in a normal tone of voice, facing the patient so the ECG technician can observe their facial expression. Depending on the degree of visual impairment the patient may not be able to see gestures or materials, so alternate forms of materials (braille handouts or enlarged text) or manipulatives must be considered. The field of vision may be impaired so that the patient sees shapes or has better vision in some areas than others, and the ECG technician should try to position herself or himself for the patient's advantage. The ECG technician should also announce his or her presence, explain actions and movement ("I'm putting the ECG supplies on the counter"), announce position ("I'm at your right side") and always tell the patient if intending to touch the patient ("I'm going to be putting stickers on your chest").

COMMUNICATION TECHNIQUES FOR INDIVIDUALS WITH INTELLECTUAL DISABILITY

Communicating with patients who are **intellectually disabled** can be challenging, and patients may have very different and individual responses, so observation of the patient must serve as a guide. Patients may be apprehensive and frightened, so the ECG technician should maintain a friendly, normal tone of voice and should speak with the patient often to establish rapport, even if the response is not clear. The ECG technician should always ask the patient before touching his or her things. Initiating communication by talking about familiar things (family, pictures, the past) may be comforting for the patient. If responses are unclear or inappropriate, the ECG technician can say, "I'm sorry, I didn't understand that," but should not laugh or indicate frustration.

COMMUNICATION TECHNIQUES WHEN ASSESSING UNDERSTANDING

Communication techniques used when assessing patient's understanding include the following:

- **Reflection**: Referring to both the meaning of the patient's words and the emotions. If a patient states, "I understand what I am supposed to do during the stress test," a reflecting question might be, "You feel confident that you know what will be required of you during the stress test?"
- **Restatement**: Restating or paraphrasing something a patient said, such as, "I've been having dizzy spells for two weeks." Restatement might be, "You've been having dizzy spells for two weeks."
- **Clarification**: Asking for more information. If a patient states, "I haven't been feeling well," a clarifying question might be, "What exactly do you mean when you say you haven't been feeling well?"
- **Feedback**: Responding to something a patient has said or done, letting them know that the message/information was received. For example, "You have kept very accurate records of your blood pressure and pulse."

INTERNAL AND EXTERNAL DISTRACTIONS THAT DISRUPT COMMUNICATION CYCLE

Distractions (interference) that disrupt the communication cycle include:

- **Internal**: The communicator's or recipient's emotional status, such as increased anxiety or anger, can negatively impact communication. Biases, prejudices, and belief systems may also interfere with a person's ability to attend to the ideas of another person. Pain and hunger can be so distracting that the person is unable to focus on communication. When under stress, the brain may process information differently, interfering with comprehension.
- **External**: Noise in the environment (conversation, traffic, alarms, air conditioning) can make it hard for some people to hear clearly, especially those with hearing impairment, and may make concentration difficult. Additionally, people may find noise very stressful to the point that they have difficulty thinking. Other environmental factors, such as extremes of heat or cold, may cause physical discomfort that interferes with the ability to communicate.

PROFESSIONAL BEHAVIOR IN THERAPEUTIC RELATIONSHIPS
MAINTAINING PROFESSIONAL BEHAVIOR IN THERAPEUTIC RELATIONSHIPS

The patient may share confidential information with the ECG technician, which makes the patient vulnerable. At the beginning of a therapeutic relationship, the ECG technician is responsible for establishing:

- Trust
- Clear, identifiable boundaries
- Mutual expectations
- Confidentiality ground rules

Respond to the patient's needs, but pursue the treatment objectives established by the doctor foremost. Demonstrate acceptance, humor, and compassion to the patient, but keep an appropriate emotional and physical distance. Limit patient contact to assisting with medical procedures, bookings, and casual conversation. It is unprofessional conduct to date or befriend patients, or give them insider information. Remember, the primary purpose of the interaction is to be therapeutic to the patient. Stay alert for:

- Inappropriate emotions imposed on another person (transference and countertransference)
- Conflict of interest (using the relationship for personal gain)

At the end of a therapeutic relationship, arrange a monitoring schedule, so that the patient is not lost to follow-up.

INTERPERSONAL SKILLS

The ECG technician must interact with colleagues, patients, families, insurance personnel, and salespeople, among others, so **interpersonal skills** (qualities and behaviors one utilizes when interacting with others) are essential. The ECG technician serves as a liaison among different parties (such as the physician and patient) and must appear friendly, cooperative, and empathetic, being especially sensitive to the needs of patients and family members, who are often anxious. The ECG technician should utilize active listening, paying attention to not only the spoken words, but also nonverbal communication and should ensure that personal nonverbal communication is appropriate. The ECG technician should understand conflict resolution and should avoid passing judgement without understanding all aspects of a problem. The ECG technician should value teamwork and model collaboration, showing respect for the opinions of others and providing positive feedback. The ECG technician should also model a positive attitude toward work, colleagues, and patients/families.

Obtain and Interpret Patient Vital Signs

STABLE VITAL SIGNS

Stable vital signs (those maintained within the normal range for the individual's age) indicate good health (homeostasis). Ill or injured patients have vital signs outside the normal range. The severity of the illness or injury is often indicated by the variability of vital sign measurements. Wide variations mean the patient is unstable. Their vital signs should be checked every five minutes. For stable patients, vital signs can be checked less frequently, depending on the circumstance. The following parameters are considered vital signs:

- Pulse
- Respiration rate
- Blood pressure
- Oxygen saturation
- Temperature

> **Review Video: Vital Signs and How to Check Them**
> Visit mometrix.com/academy and enter code: 330799

PULSE

The pulse is a surge of blood through an artery that occurs when the heart contracts (during systole). The key **pulse points** are:

- **Apical**: Over the heart
- **Brachial**: In the elbow bend (most common site for palpation in children under 1 year)
- **Carotid**: In the neck (for pulse checks in unconscious patients; be sure to only palpate one side at a time to maintain perfusion to the brain)
- **Dorsalis pedis**: On top of the foot
- **Facial**: On the jaw under the mouth
- **Femoral**: In the groin (for pulse checks in unconscious patients)
- **Popliteal**: On the back of the knee
- **Posterior tibial**: On the back of the ankle
- **Radial**: On the anterior wrist below the thumb (most common site for palpation in patients older than 1 year)
- **Temporal**: On the temple
- **Ulnar**: On the anterior wrist below the little finger

Pulse **rate** varies by age:

Normal Resting Pulse Rate	Age
60–100 beats per minute	Adult
80–100 beats per minute	Child
100 beats per minute	Toddler
100–140 beats per minute	Infant under one year
up to 150 beats per minute	Newborn (neonate)

DISTAL PULSE AND PULSE DEFICIT

If a **distal pulse** cannot be felt in the patient's limbs, first utilize a doppler machine to find the pulse. If it still cannot be found, find the apical pulse in the chest. Count to the 5th rib space in the middle of the left side of the chest or midclavicular line. If the apical pulse is regular, count for 30 seconds and record the reading. If the apical pulse is irregular, count for a full minute and record the reading. Report an irregular pulse to the doctor to evaluate for possible pulse deficit. A **pulse deficit** occurs when the radial pulse in the wrist is slower than the apical pulse in the chest. A pulse deficit can indicate that the patient has weak heart contractions, which fail to transmit beats to the peripheral arterial system.

TACHYCARDIA AND BRADYCARDIA

Tachycardia is a pulse rate over 100 beats per minute, which may be caused by anxiety, fear, stress, pneumonia, anemia, low blood pressure, dehydration, fever, infection, hyperthyroidism, and heart conditions.

Bradycardia is a resting heart rate less than 60 beats per minute, which may be caused by a heart attack (MI), hypothermia, heat exhaustion, obstructive jaundice, skull fracture, malnutrition, hypothyroidism, and many adverse drug reactions. Olympic athletes may have bradycardia because their hearts are extremely efficient.

MEASURING RESPIRATIONS

Measuring respirations is done to assess the number of times per minute the patient breathes. Typically, when a person is made aware of their breathing, they do not breathe deeply or regularly. Do not tell the patient when measuring the respiration rate, as it may make them aware of their breathing and produce an inaccurate result. The ideal time to measure the patient's respiration rate is after checking the patient's pulse. Count the number of times the patient breathes, counting one rise and fall of the chest wall as one respiration. Count the number of breaths for one minute, noting the depth of the breath and any use of accessory muscles. Record the respiratory rate on the patient's chart.

INDICATIONS OF ABNORMAL RESPIRATIONS

The normal range for respiratory rate for adults is 12–20 breaths per minute. A number of factors may affect the rate of the patient's breathing. The patient may breathe more slowly if resting or if he is positioned on his back. Certain narcotics may also depress the respiratory drive, resulting in fewer breaths per minute. A rapid respiration rate may be caused by increased activity, pain, or stress. An elevated temperature or an infection may cause the patient's respiratory rate to be quicker. Other conditions, such as respiratory distress, fluid overload, or a heart attack, may also cause an elevated respiratory rate.

BLOOD PRESSURE

Increased blood pressure contributes to stroke and heart disease. Low blood pressure is associated with shock, trauma, bleeding, or severe infection. Blood pressure is defined by the following parameters:

- Normal adult blood pressure: Systole <120 mmHg, diastole <80 mmHg
- Prehypertension: Systole 120–129, diastole <80
- Hypertension stage 1: Systole 130–139, diastole 80–89
- Hypertension stage 2: Systole ≥140, diastole ≥90
- Hypotension (low blood pressure): 90/50 or less

False BP reading can occur from the following:

- **Incorrect cuff size**: If the patient is obese, use a thigh cuff on the upper arm. Bariatric blood pressure cuffs also exist. If the patient is a child, use a pediatric cuff.
- **Deflating the cuff more rapidly** than 2–3 mmHg per second can inhibit the ability to accurately record both systole and diastole.
- **Venous congestion** makes it difficult to hear the blood pressure sounds. Elevating the patient's arm after positioning the cuff but before inflating it can decrease venous congestion.
- Loud **environmental noises**
- **Operator error**

OBTAINING A MANUAL BLOOD PRESSURE

When obtaining **a** manual blood pressure, a correctly sized cuff is essential. The cuff width should be 40% of the circumference (or 20% wider than the diameter) of the middle of the limb to which the blood pressure cuff will be applied. The bladder (which fills with air as the cuff is inflated) should circle at least 80% of the limb and the cuff width (when used on the upper arm) should cover two-thirds of the length of the upper arm. Small or extra-large blood pressure cuffs may be indicated. Cuffs should not be applied to a limb receiving IV fluids or one that is traumatized. The forearm (or leg) should be at heart level and the hand turned up if using an arm. Procedure:

1. Palpate brachial or peripheral artery, deflate cuff completely, and apply snugly to the site (two fingers should be able to fit between the cuff and arm), aligning the centering arrows correctly or centering the bladder over the artery. Cuff should be one-inch above site of arterial pulsation (popliteal or antecubital).
2. Inflate bladder and increase pressure to about 30 mmHg above anticipated base or 30 mmHg above where pulse is no longer palpable.
3. Slowly release air and note when heart sound appears (systolic) and when it disappears (diastolic).
4. Record BP reading.

ANEROID SPHYGMOMANOMETER

Blood pressure is measured as systolic and diastolic pressure by means of a stethoscope and an **aneroid sphygmomanometer** (portable blood pressure cuff). For example, if the reading is 120/80 mmHg, 120 is the systole, and 80 is the diastole. The first Korotkoff sound the ECG technician hears ('lub') is the systole; the last Korotkoff sound ('dub') is the diastole.

> **Review Video: Diastolic vs Systolic**
> Visit mometrix.com/academy and enter code: 898934

OXYGEN SATURATION

Pulse oximetry non-invasively measures a patient's oxyhemoglobin (oxygen saturation) level using a small clip-like device with a light that measures the oxygen saturation of the site it is attached to. This is a painless method of monitoring an individual's respiratory status and perfusion over a period of time when attached continuously, or in a single moment as part of a physical assessment. Attach the oximeter sensor to one of the patient's first three fingers (index, middle or ring). If the patient's hands are damaged, use a toe or earlobe. Consider using the forehead, nose, or other parts of the foot only as a last resort. Normal range should fall between 95% and 100%, although patients with certain conditions, such as COPD, may have a chronically lower saturation. If a patient's oxygen saturation falls below normal range persistently, the ECG technician must inform the doctor that the patient is hypoxic. Many pulse oximeters also measure the patient's heart rate at the same time. A pulse oximeter is not accurate if the patient is very anemic, has poor circulation (due to being cold or having vascular abnormalities), is edematous, moves a lot, or wears artificial nails or very dark nail polish. Adjust the room temperature, lighting, and move electronic equipment to get a good reading.

BODY TEMPERATURE

A live patient's body temperature is measured to determine if he or she is storing and releasing heat properly, to detect abnormally high or low body temperatures, and to assess the effectiveness of some types of medications. The coroner measures temperature to determine time of death. Adult normal temperature ranges are as follows:

- Normal range: 97–99 °F (36.1–37.2 °C)
- Hypothermia (too cold): <95 °F (<35 °C)
- Pyrexia (fever): >100.4 °F (>38 °C)
- Hyperpyrexia (lethal fever): >106.7 °F (>41.5 °C)

Temperature is at its lowest around 4:00 a.m. and highest around 6:00 p.m. Temperature spikes often occur after meals. Ovulation in women creates a temperature rise of 0.5–1.0 °F when measured before arising from bed in the morning (basal body temperature). Individual temperature differences in healthy people are due to the rate of metabolism. Patients with hypothyroidism tend to be cold. Body temperature differs at different sites. Normal oral temperature is 98.6 °F, while rectal temperature is 0.5–1.0 °F higher than oral temperature, and axillary temperature is usually 0.5–1.0 °F lower than oral temperature. Do not take the patient's oral temperature for 30 minutes after eating or drinking, as it will be raised with hot food, and lowered with cold drinks.

ENSURING PATIENT SAFETY DURING PROCEDURES

Measures to ensure patient safety during procedures include the following:

- **Fall risk**: Be aware of a patient's fall risk status, which is generally posted in or near their room. Consider possible vision impairments and ensure easy access to glasses if applicable. Understand medications that may influence fall risk, such as sedatives and blood pressure (BP) medications. After capturing the patient's ECG, ensure that fall precautions remain in or are returned to their place. Return the side table to an easy-to-access position and ask the patient if there is anything that is needed before leaving the room. In the case of cardiac stress testing, assist the patient to step onto and off of the treadmill. Ask the patient before the procedure about a history of falls, dizziness, or mobility issues that may impact testing. Ensure that handrails are within easy reach, and keep a chair near the treadmill in case the patient needs to quickly sit down. Monitor the patient continuously during stress testing.
- **Call bell access**: Instruct patients in call bell use and ensure that it is within reach if the patient is left alone for any period of time. If the patient has limited mobility, place the call bell in the patient's hand or attach it where it is easily reachable. If there is no call bell, instruct patients on alternative methods of calling for assistance, such as raising a hand to indicate distress or communicating verbally.
- **Bed side rails**: An upper side rail on the side that the technician is working can be lowered while applying electrodes, but then, once the electrodes are placed, the upper side rails are typically raised, but the lower side rails are not raised unless ordered to do so by the physician. Patients should not be left unattended when an upper side rail is lowered.

Patient Preparation for Stress Testing

PREPARING PATIENTS FOR STRESS TESTING

Patients scheduled for a **stress test** should understand what the procedure entails, about how long it will take, and any post-test instructions. They should also be assured that they will be continuously monitored and will be advised to notify healthcare professionals if any adverse effects, such as chest pain, weakness, or dizziness, occur during testing. Instructions may vary somewhat but typically include:

- Do not smoke and do not eat or drink anything with caffeine (e.g., chocolate, soda, tea, coffee, Anacin, Excedrin) for 24 hours prior to the test.
- Avoid eating and drinking for 4–6 hours before the test except for small amounts of water with medications.
- Wear clothing that is loose fitting and comfortable.
- Avoid performing strenuous exercise on the day of the test.
- Depending on the type of test, you may need to discontinue some medications. For example, if the patient is to receive dobutamine during testing, beta-blockers may be withheld.
- During the test, you will need to remove clothing any above the waist, although women may wear a sports bra, and a gown will be provided.
- The skin is prepped for electrode placement on the chest. Hair may be removed by shaving or clipping for males.

TYPES OF STRESS TESTS

TREADMILL AND STATIONARY BIKE

Exercise (e.g., treadmill, stationary bicycle) stress testing is used to evaluate heart function under physical stress. Baseline ECG, BP, oxygen saturation, and heart rate measurements are recorded and are continually monitored during the procedure. The patient walks on the treadmill or rides a cycle ergometer for the test. The **Bruce protocol** is usually used, which comprises seven 3-minute phases of increasing speed and incline of the treadmill or effort on the cycle until the patient reaches maximal effort or experiences adverse symptoms. Patients begin with speed of 1.7 mph and an incline of 10% and this slowly increases to a speed of 6 mph and an incline of 22%. A **modified Bruce protocol** may be used for elderly patients or those with heart failure. It maintains 1.7 mph for the first three phases and begins with no incline. The stress test ends with a slowdown period of 3–6 minutes. The patient is monitored until the heart rate, BP, and ECG return to baseline. The test is terminated if the patient develops angina, severe shortness of breath, leg fatigue, dizziness, significant ECG changes (arrhythmias, ST segment depression >2 mm), or an abnormal BP response.

Safety, Compliance, and
Coordinated Patient Care

PHARMACOLOGIC

Pharmacologic stress tests are used for patients with exercise intolerance, to assess cardiac risk preoperatively, and to evaluate myocardial perfusion. Types of tests include the following:

- **Vasodilator test:** Adenosine, regadenoson, or dipyridamole are administered IV to dilate the coronary arteries. Tests with adenosine and regadenoson typically take 10 to 15 minutes and usually do not require a reversal agent, whereas, with dipyridamole, the test takes 20 to 30 minutes and aminophylline is required at the completion of the test to reverse its effects. The vasodilator test is usually combined with nuclear imaging (by single-photon emission computed tomography/positron emission tomography, stress magnetic resonance imaging [MRI]) to detect blood flow since the blood flow decreases with stenosis. Common adverse effects include flushing, chest discomfort, bronchospasm, hypotension, and headache.
- **Dobutamine test:** If vasodilators are contraindicated, this test uses dobutamine, a beta-1 adrenergic agonist, to increase the heart rate and cardiac contractility. The patient is monitored with ECG and echocardiogram during the test. Dobutamine is administered IV in increasing dosages every 3 minutes, five times. The test is continued until the target heart rate is achieved (i.e., 85% of the maximum predicted heart rate) or adverse effects, such as significant ischemia, chest pain, nausea, or arrhythmias, occur. If the heart rate is excessive or if the patient develops palpitations, esmolol is used as a reversal agent.

STRESS ECHOCARDIOGRAPHY, NUCLEAR STRESS TEST/MYOCARDIAL PERFUSION IMAGING, AND CARDIOPULMONARY EXERCISE TESTING

Stress echocardiography may be used with suspected coronary artery disease, to assess the heart after a myocardial infarction, and to evaluate heart valve disease. A baseline echocardiogram is obtained, and then the patient carries out the prescribed exercise or pharmacologic stressor followed by a poststress echocardiogram. The images from the prestress period and the poststress period are compared.

Nuclear stress test/myocardial perfusion imaging is used to assess the flow of blood in the heart muscle at rest and during stress. A radioactive tracer (e.g., technetium-99m or thallium-201) is administered IV, and then images are taken while the patient is at rest and again after a period of exercise or pharmacologic stress.

Cardiopulmonary exercise testing assesses exercise capacity and oxygen consumption. It is used to distinguish cardiac limitations from pulmonary ones. The patient exercises (with a treadmill or cycle ergometer) while the ECG, BP, oxygen consumption, carbon dioxide production, and ventilation are monitored and measured.

STRESS CARDIAC MRI, STRESS POSITRON EMISSION TOMOGRAPHY, AND PACING STRESS TEST

Stress cardiac MRI is used to evaluate myocardial perfusion. ECG electrodes are placed on the chest so that the MRI images can sync with the heartbeat. Images are initially taken at rest, and then pharmacologic stress is induced with a vasodilator or dobutamine. When stress is achieved, a gadolinium contrast agent is administered IV and further images are immediately taken. The pharmacologic agent is stopped, and the patient is monitored until recovery; then, another set of resting images is taken.

Stress positron emission tomography is used to assess myocardial perfusion and myocardial viability. A radioactive tracer (rubidium-82, ammonia-13, or fludeoxyglucose-18) is administered IV, and baseline myocardial perfusion images are taken. Then, the patient receives pharmacologic stress (with a vasodilator). When stress reaches its peak, another dose of the radioactive tracer is administered and images are taken. After the vasodilator is stopped and the patient recovers, additional images may be taken in some cases.

The **pacing stress test** is used for patients with an implanted pacemaker, which is programmed to increase the heart rate to the target rate of 85% of the age-predicted maximum heart rate or to the rate at which signs of ischemia occur. Continuous ECG, BP, and oxygen saturation monitoring is done throughout the procedure.

Ambulatory Monitoring

TYPES OF HOLTER MONITORS

The Holter monitor is used for ambulatory heart monitoring. There are three basic types:

- **Traditional:** Has electrodes (3-, 5-, or 12-lead) applied to the skin and wires leading to a recording device that is usually worn about the waist. Recordings are continuous. Monitors for 24 to 48 hours. Lead placement is like standard ECGs. A symptom log is required, and some monitors have a button to press if an adverse event occurs.
- **Patch**: Patch monitors, such as the Zio Patch, are single-use devices without external wires and can extend the cardiac monitoring time to 14 days. Applied to the left chest (two finger-widths below the clavicle and to the left of the sternum, at or above the level of the breast). Recordings are continuous. Patch monitors have a button to press if an adverse event occurs. Symptom logs are often recommended.
- **Event recorder** (lead or patch): Event recorders, such as BardyDx CAM, record only when activated by pushing a button and may be used from 30 days up to months. A symptom log is often recommended. Used for intermittent arrhythmias.

Bluetooth-enabled Holter monitors (lead or patch) transmit data in real time and can record cardiac data for up to 30 days.

PATIENT INSTRUCTIONS FOR LEAD- AND PATCH-TYPE HOLTER MONITORS

Holter monitor leads are applied by healthcare providers, but patients may be instructed to apply patch monitors. The skin should be clean and dry before application, and hair should be removed or trimmed. Additional instructions are dependent on the type of monitor.

For lead monitors:

- Keep electrodes dry: Avoid swimming, showering, and bathing.
- Wear loose-fitting clothing to avoid pulling on the wires.
- Avoid lotions, oils, or powders on the chest.
- Avoid high-voltage areas (e.g., microwaves, metal detectors, computed tomography scans, x-rays) and MRIs, and do not use electric blankets.
- Press the button on the monitor and record adverse events (e.g., dyspnea, chest pain, palpitations, skipped beats, dizziness) in the symptom log.

For patch monitors:

- Avoid showering for 24 hours after placement and avoid any direct water or submergence of monitor during showering and bathing.
- Avoid activities that cause excessive sweating.
- Avoid MRIs (monitor contains metals).
- Report itching or skin irritation from the adhesive holding monitor in place.
- Press the button to indicate adverse events and record in the symptom log if so directed.
- Avoid placing an electric blanket directly over the patch because heat may loosen the adhesive.
- Remove the patch monitor as directed: Wash hands, lift the outer edges away from the skin, pulling sideways rather than straight up. Gently wash the skin with soap and water. Apply moisturizer if the skin gets irritated.

Utilization of Electronic Health Records

REVIEWING THE PATIENT'S ELECTRONIC HEALTH RECORD

Key patient information from the health record should be reviewed by the ECG technician:

- Demographics: Name, date of birth, medical record number, room number (for inpatients), and physician's order for the ECG and reason for the test
- Medical history and cardiac risk factors, such as a history of heart disease or hypertension
- Previous ECGs: Review and compare if available
- Vital signs and oxygen saturation
- Conditions that may affect ECG waveforms: Chronic obstructive pulmonary disease, asthma, pulmonary embolism, neuromuscular disorders (e.g., Parkinson's disease, intention tremors, muscular dystrophy, electrolyte imbalances)
- Medications that may affect ECG waveforms: Beta-blockers (bradycardia), calcium channel blockers (slow conduction), digoxin (ST depression and T wave changes), antiarrhythmic drugs (prolong the QT interval), loop diuretics (hypokalemia causing U waves and ventricular arrhythmias), antidepressants and antipsychotics (prolong the QT interval)
- Presence of implantable devices, such as a pacemaker or implantable cardioverter-defibrillator or deep brain stimulators (may cause electrical interference)
- Surgical history that may affect electrode placement: Chest trauma, bilateral mastectomy, limb amputation
- Special considerations that may affect electrode placement: Pregnancy, obesity, pediatric patient, contractures

BASIC ELEMENTS AND PROCESSES RELATED TO ELECTRONIC HEALTH RECORDS

To **document an ECG** in electronic medical records/electronic health records, most systems have structured fields (i.e., designated areas in which information is entered in text). Demographic information, such as a patient's name, date of birth, medical record numbers, is usually entered into the fields. Other information may be entered through selections from drop-down menus—for example, the ECG type; the reason for the ECG; the date; the patient's positioning; electrode placement; skin preparation; patient tolerance; and technical issues, such as signal quality, and the need for repeated attempts. If drop-down menus are not available, then this information would be entered into the notes in text. Generally, ECG technicians are not allowed to interpret ECG findings, but (if allowed) they may indicate basic findings, such as bradycardia/tachycardia or atrial fibrillation. The ECG technician should also record whether the ECG was stat or routine and how the ECG report was transmitted. Some electronic medical record/electronic health record systems allow for automatic transmission of ECGs, but other systems may require that the ECG be uploaded to the system—protocols may vary.

Signs and Symptoms of Cardiopulmonary Compromise

SINGLE-RESCUER CPR FOR ADULT VICTIM

Only perform CPR on a patient with cardiac arrest, who is unresponsive, with no pulse or breathing. After calling for help and/or activating a code blue per facility protocol, don gloves, if possible. Place the patient supine on the floor. Look, listen, and feel for the patient's breathing and pulse. If there is no pulse, immediately start chest compressions at a 30:2 compression-breath ratio. If there is a pulse, but no breathing, open the patient's airway by inclining the head back and raising the chin. Place a resuscitation mouthpiece into the patient's mouth. Pinch the nose closed. Inflate the lungs with two breaths. Observe the chest's rise and fall. Check the carotid pulse after administering the rescue breaths. If the pulse has been lost, kneel beside the patient. Landmark the xiphoid process at the end of the sternum (breastbone), where the ribs meet. Place palms over the breastbone. Compress 30 times, followed by two breaths. After four cycles, check the carotid pulse again. Pulse checks should never be longer than 10 seconds. Continue until the patient regains a pulse/breathing or until a rescuer with higher training arrives to provide relief. Discard the mouthpiece. Document CPR in the patient's chart.

AED

An **automated external defibrillator (AED)** can revive an individual that is in specific types of cardiac arrest, providing it is applied within four minutes and damage is not extensive. Continue CPR until the unit is charged. The patient must be on a flat, dry surface. Connect the pads of the AED to the patient, as illustrated on the unit. Press the "analyze" button first for a readout, to ensure the unit is ready and electroshock is appropriate. Announce, "stay clear of the patient" while the AED is analyzing the patient's rhythm. Restart chest compressions if defibrillation is contraindicated (in the case of asystole or ventricular tachycardia with a palpable pulse). The unit indicates by tone or light that it is ready to shock the patient. The AED display shows when defibrillation occurs. Check the pulse after the third shock. If there is a pulse, check the airway, breathing, and circulation and move the patient into recovery position. If there is no pulse, continue CPR. The defibrillator will continue to provide instructions through this process. When the defibrillator announces that it is analyzing, the patient must not be touched. Continue CPR as directed by the AED. The unit indicates when to stop defibrillation.

SYNCOPE

Syncope is characterized by fainting due to a temporary loss of consciousness caused by a disruption in the blood flow to the brain. The insufficiency of blood results in a lack of oxygen in the brain. When the patient falls into horizontal position, blood flow to the brain is restored and the problem corrects itself. After a patient regains consciousness, place the patient in recovery position. Alert the doctor/nurse if they did not witness the event. Syncope may result from the following:

- Emotional stress/fear
- Physical pain
- Standing in one position for too long
- Overheating
- Dehydration
- Exhaustion
- Rapid changes in blood pressure
- Heart disease
- Neurological disorders
- Lung disease
- Adverse reaction to medication

If syncope occurs with exercise or is associated with irregularities in heart rhythm, it can indicate a serious health problem. Sharp muscle contractions called myoclonic jerks may occur with syncope. This is not true seizure activity. Bradycardia and increased vagal tone are often seen in cases of syncope.

CHEST PAIN

Chest pain may indicate **angina** (pain from temporary constriction/blockage of blood flow in the coronary arteries) or a heart attack (pain caused by blockage of blood flow to the heart muscle because of a blood clot (most common) or hemorrhage, resulting in the death of heart tissue). Heart problems in children are often associated with congenital heart disease. Geriatric and female patients may not have chest pain with a heart attack. Make note of the following:

- Character, location, and severity of the pain.
- Radiation of pain to the neck, jaw, arms, back, jaw, and/or stomach.
- Shortness of breath at rest, with exertion, or worsening when lying flat.
- Cold, clammy skin is common with a heart attack.
- Note BP, pulse (rapid, irregular, slow), and respirations.
- Note nausea and/or vomiting and dizziness/lightheadedness.

ANGINA PECTORIS (STABLE)

Impairment of blood flow through the coronary arteries leads to ischemia of the cardiac muscle and **angina pectoris**—pain that may occur in the sternum, chest, neck, arms (especially the left arm), or back. The pain frequently occurs with crushing pain substernally, radiating down the left arm or both arms, although this type of pain is more common in males than females, whose symptoms may appear less acute and may include nausea, shortness of breath, and fatigue. Elderly or diabetic patients may also have pain in their arms, no pain at all (silent ischemia), or weakness and numbness in both arms.

Stable angina episodes usually last for <5 minutes and are fairly predictable, exercise-induced episodes caused by atherosclerotic lesions blocking >75% of the lumen of the affected coronary artery. Precipitating events include exercise, a decrease in the environmental temperature, heavy eating, strong emotions (such as fright or anger), or exertion, including coitus. Stable angina episodes usually resolve in less than 5 minutes by decreasing the activity level and administering sublingual nitroglycerin. Provide supportive care, oxygen, and assist the patient to take nitroglycerin if available.

ANGINA PECTORIS (UNSTABLE, VARIANT/PRINZMETAL'S)

Unstable angina (also known as preinfarction or crescendo angina) is a progression of coronary artery disease, and it occurs when there is a change in the pattern of stable angina. The pain may increase, may not respond to a single nitroglycerin dose, and may persist for >5 minutes. Usually pain is more frequent, lasts longer, and may occur at rest when sitting or lying down. Unstable angina may indicate a rupture of an atherosclerotic plaque and the beginning of thrombus formation, so it should always be treated as a medical emergency with rapid transport because it may indicate a myocardial infarction.

Variant angina (also known as **Prinzmetal's angina**) results from spasms of the coronary arteries. It can be associated with or without atherosclerotic plaques and is often related to smoking, alcohol, or illicit stimulants. Variant angina frequently occurs cyclically at the same time each day and often while the person is at rest. Nitroglycerin or calcium channel blockers are used for treatment.

MANAGEMENT OF A PATIENT WITH ANGINA

Management of a patient with angina begins with a thorough assessment by a medical professional, primary and secondary survey, and use of the OPQRST and SAMPLE methods of history taking. Patients are often very frightened, so the ECG technician can provide support and reassurance. The patient should be placed in the semi-Fowler's position, especially if he or she is experiencing shortness of breath, and the oxygen saturation should be monitored. Respiratory compromise may require supplemental oxygen, bag-mask ventilation (BVM) assistance, PEEP, CPAP/BiPAP, manually triggered ventilators (MTVs), or automatic transport ventilators (ATVs). This support must be provided by the physician and nursing staff.

Pharmacological interventions (assist the patient with medication administration, or administer the medication according to protocol) may include aspirin, nitroglycerin, or oral glucose. All patients with chest pain should result in escalation to a physician because even mild chest discomfort may indicate that the patient is having a heart attack, especially in older patients and female patients, who often have atypical symptoms.

MYOCARDIAL INFARCTION

Myocardial infarction (also referred to as an MI or heart attack) may occur after an episode of unstable angina caused by a rupture of an atherosclerotic plaque and thrombosis associated with coronary artery spasm, but it may also result from vasoconstriction, acute blood loss, decreased oxygen, and ingestion of cocaine. Symptoms may vary considerably, with males having the more "classic" symptom of a sudden onset of crushing chest pain. Elderly and diabetic patients may complain primarily of weakness. Symptoms include the following:

- Angina with pain in the chest that may radiate to the neck or arms, crushing pain, tightness (often more than 30 minutes and unrelieved by rest or nitroglycerin).
- Hypertension or hypotension.
- Palpitations, tachycardia, bradycardia, and dysrhythmias.
- Dyspnea.
- ECG changes (ST segment and T-wave changes), tachycardia, bradycardia, and dysrhythmias.
- Pulmonary edema, peripheral edema, weak/absent peripheral pulses.
- Nausea and vomiting.
- Pallor, cold and clammy skin, diaphoresis.
- Neurological/psychological disturbances: Anxiety, light-headedness, headache, visual abnormalities, slurred speech, and fear.

If a patient is suspected to be having a heart attack the ECG technician must immediately call a Code Blue or Rapid Response (per facility protocol) and initiate CPR if the patient loses consciousness while awaiting assistance.

> **Review Video: Myocardial Infarction**
> Visit mometrix.com/academy and enter code: 148923

ECG Acquisition

Basic Anatomy and Physiology of the Heart

CARDIOVASCULAR SYSTEM

The cardiovascular system controls blood flow throughout the body and to the tissues, controls gas exchange (carbon dioxide and oxygen) by transporting oxygenated blood from the lungs, serves as a reservoir for blood, maintains blood pH through a buffer system, responds to infections, and facilitates coagulation (blood clotting). The cardiovascular system has the following components:

- **Heart**: The heart has four chambers, two upper (right atrium, left atrium) and two lower (right ventricle and left ventricle). The heart muscle receives blood from four major coronary arteries (right, left main, left anterior descending, and left circumflex) and their branches, and then distributes blood via the aorta and pulmonary arteries.
- **Vessels**: The venous system includes veins, venules, and venous capillaries and returns blood back to the heart via the inferior and superior vena cava. The arterial system, (including the coronary arteries) branches from the aorta after it leaves the heart and includes arteries, arterioles, and arterial capillaries.
- **Blood**: Blood consists of red blood cells (erythrocytes), white blood cells (leukocytes including monocytes, lymphocytes, basophils, neutrophils, and eosinophils), platelets (thrombocytes), and plasma, the liquid portion of the blood (which contains clotting factors). Blood carries oxygen from the lungs and distributes it to the rest of the body.

The cardiovascular system is responsible for oxygenation of cells, perfusion (carrying of blood with oxygen, glucose, and nutrients to cells) and removing waste products, such as carbon dioxide.

> **Review Video: Cardiovascular System**
> Visit mometrix.com/academy and enter code: 376581

ANATOMY OF THE HEART

The human heart is about the size of a fist and weighs 7–15 ounces. It is located in the middle of the chest, behind the sternum, and leans slightly left. The heart is covered by a double-layered membrane called the **pericardium**. The outer layer, called the parietal pericardium, is fibrous and surrounds the roots of the major blood vessels of the heart. The inner layer, called the visceral pericardium, is attached to and covers the heart muscle. The two layers of membrane are separated by fluid. The heart itself has **four connecting chambers**. The two upper chambers are the **right atria and left atria**; the lower chambers are the **left ventricle and right ventricle**. The left and right atria and the left and right ventricle are separated by a muscular structure called the septum.

> **Review Video: Heart Anatomy and Physiology**
> Visit mometrix.com/academy and enter code: 569724

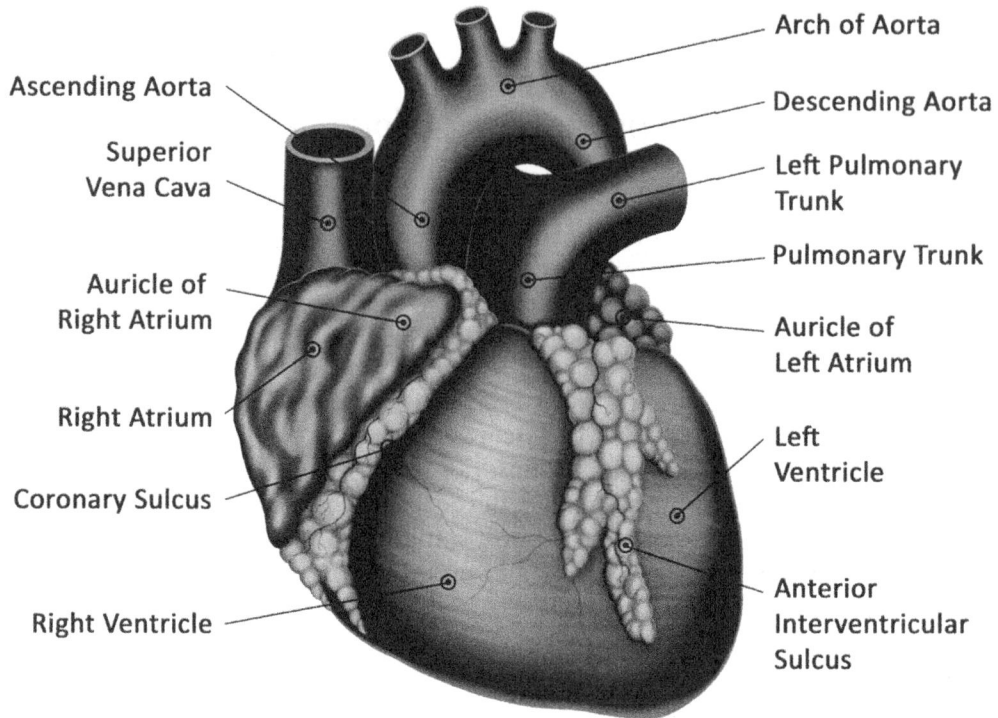

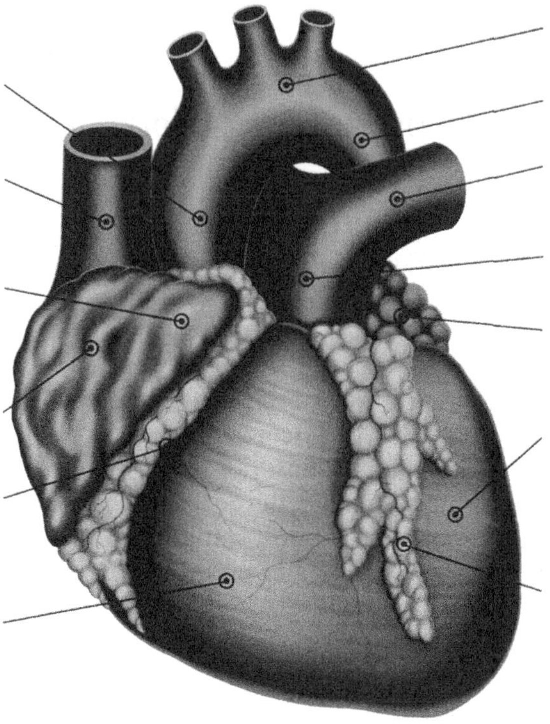
Ascending Aorta
Superior Vena Cava
Auricle of Right Atrium
Right Atrium
Coronary Sulcus
Right Ventricle
Arch of Aorta
Descending Aorta
Left Pulmonary Trunk
Pulmonary Trunk
Auricle of Left Atrium
Left Ventricle
Anterior Interventricular Sulcus

HEART'S CONDUCTION SYSTEM

The **sinoatrial node (SA)** is referred to as the pacemaker of the heart because electrical impulses normally originate in the SA, within the wall of the right atrium. The SA produces electrical impulses that are transmitted to the **atrioventricular node (AV)** by specialized conducting tissue. The AV node is found between the atria and ventricles. From here, the electrical impulse is relayed down the conducting tissue called the Bundle of His. The **Bundle of His** splits into a right bundle branch (RBB) and a left bundle branch (LBB), which serve the right and left ventricles, respectively, through both sides of the intraventricular septum. The bundle branches then split to form the **Purkinje fibers**, which transmit electrical impulses to the myocardium.

Review Video: Electrical Conduction System of the Heart
Visit mometrix.com/academy and enter code: 624557

A **normal sinus rhythm** on an ECG (the expected result in a healthy individual) denotes that the electrical impulses start in the sinoatrial node (SA) first. The intrinsic rate of the SA node is 60–100 beats per minute (bpm), which reflects the normal range for an adult's pulse rate. If the SA node does not initiate the electrical impulse, the atrioventricular node (AV) can do so. However, the AV node is not as capable of increasing the heart rate, with an intrinsic rate of only 40–60 beats per minute. The patient may require a pacemaker to address the slow heart rate. All of the cells of the heart are capable of generating the electrical impulses necessary to trigger a heartbeat (automaticity). Signal conduction problems (block) can occur at any site along the conduction pathway, causing alterations in the normal rhythm (arrhythmia).

HEART VALVES AND BLOOD FLOW

Four heart valves regulate the flow of blood through the heart.

- The **tricuspid valve** controls the flow of deoxygenated blood from the right atrium to the right ventricle.
- The **pulmonary semilunar valve** controls the flow of blood from the right ventricle to the pulmonary artery. The pulmonary artery carries the blood into the lungs where it is oxygenated.
- The blood then flows through the pulmonary vein back to the heart, and the **mitral valve** controls the flow of the now oxygenated blood from the left atrium to the left ventricle.
- The **aortic semilunar valve** regulates blood flow from the left ventricle to the aorta. From the aorta, the oxygenated blood is conducted to the rest of the body. The deoxygenated blood travels through the venules, then the veins, and then the inferior vena cava and superior vena cava back to the right atrium.

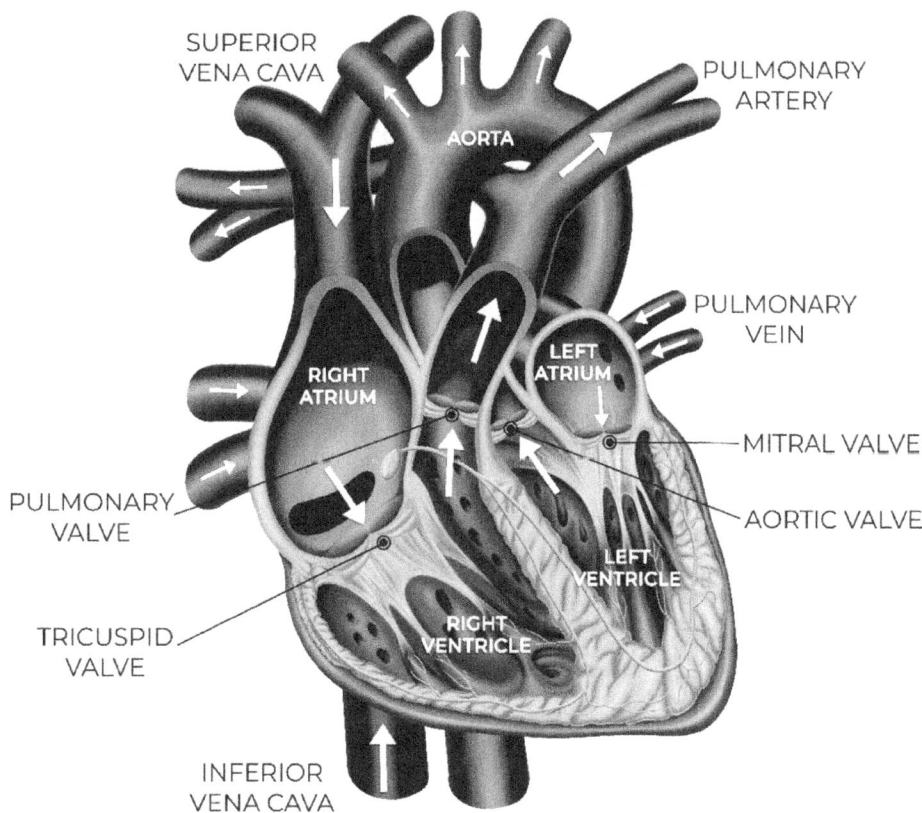

Review Video: <u>Heart Blood Flow</u>	
Visit mometrix.com/academy and enter code: 783139	

CARDIOVASCULAR DISORDERS

Cardiovascular disorders include the following:

- **Atherosclerosis**: Atherosclerosis is characterized by fatty deposits that build up inside of arteries, resulting in decreased blood flow because of narrowing and stiffening of the arteries, which in turn leads to high blood pressure and increased risk of thrombi (blood clots) and emboli (moving clots).
- **Edema**: Edema is swelling from fluid retention. Edema may occur because of heart failure (weakness of the heart muscle) that causes fluid to build up in the legs and feet and/or in the lungs (causing shortness of breath). Edema (often involving the whole body) may also occur with kidney disease and severe allergic (anaphylactic) reaction.
- **Thrombophlebitis**: Thrombophlebitis is inflammation of a vein that occurs as the result of a thrombus (blood clot) forming in the vein. The vein appears red, swollen, and tender and is at increased risk of spreading emboli to other areas of the body, such as the brain (stroke) and heart (heart attack).
- **Heart failure**: Heart failure is cardiac disease that includes disorders of contractions (systolic dysfunction) or filling (diastolic dysfunction) or both and may include pulmonary, peripheral, or systemic edema. The most common causes are coronary artery disease, systemic or pulmonary hypertension, cardiomyopathy, and valvular disorders. The incidence of chronic heart failure correlates with age. Heart failure progresses through Class I to Class IV, involving congestion in the lungs, limitations of activity, and discomfort. Uncontrolled heart failure leads to death.

Maintaining Equipment and Verifying Settings

GENERAL CONCEPTS OF ELECTROCARDIOGRAPH

An electrocardiograph machine records the heart's electrical activity on an **electrocardiogram** (ECG or ECG). The ECG monitors heart rate, patterns of heartbeats, the size and location of the chambers of the heart, and helps to diagnose heart conditions. The ECG is a non-invasive, painless, inexpensive way to determine if there is any damage to the heart muscle (myocardium) or electrical conduction system. The cardiologist uses the ECG to determine if drug therapy or pacemaker implants are having the desired effect. The P wave on an ECG corresponds to the atria contracting. The QRS complex corresponds to the ventricles contracting. The T wave is repolarization. Some conditions present via ECG based on the duration of their interval.

- Normal PR interval: 0.12 – 0.20 seconds (>0.20 seconds indicates a heart block and <0.12 may indicate disorders of excitement such as Wolff-Parkinson-White syndrome.
- Normal QRS interval: 0.08 – 0.10 seconds (>0.12 seconds indicates a widened QRS which may indicate a ventricular arrhythmia; <0.08 seconds indicates tachycardia)
- Elevated ST segment: indicates myocardial infarction (damage to the muscle of the heart due to ischemia)

For a **resting ECG**, position the patient lying down, face up. If the patient has difficulty breathing (dyspnea), prop the patient's head up with pillows. For a **stress test**, 12–15 leads are attached to the patient, who runs on a treadmill. For a **Holter monitor**, 3–5 leads are used, and the results of the ECG are recorded on a telemetry device worn around the patient's neck for 24–48 hours.

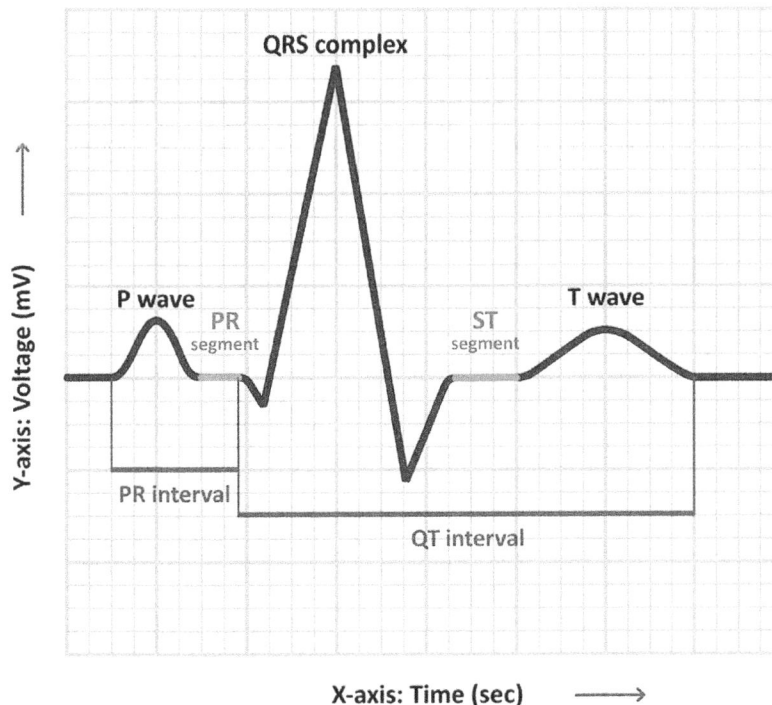

> **Review Video: ECG Rhythms – Reading the Graph**
> Visit mometrix.com/academy and enter code: 872282

45

SECTION OF HEART MONITORED IN EACH ECG LEAD

An ECG lead is the wire and electrode that connects the patient to the electrocardiograph machine (also abbreviated ECG). A standard 12-lead ECG actually has only 10 wires and electrodes, which record 12 electrical vectors:

- **Unipolar Leads**:
  - Augmented Vector Right (AVR) [right atrial view]
  - Augmented Vector Left (AVL) [lateral view]
  - Augmented Vector Foot (AVF) [inferior view]
  - Precordial chest lead V1 [anterior view]
  - Precordial chest lead V2 [anterior view]
  - Precordial chest lead V3 [septal view]
  - Precordial chest lead V4 [septal view]
  - Precordial chest lead V5 [lateral view]
  - Precordial chest lead V6 [lateral view]

- **Bipolar Leads**:
  - Limb lead I [lateral view]
  - Limb lead II [inferior view]
  - Limb lead III [inferior view]

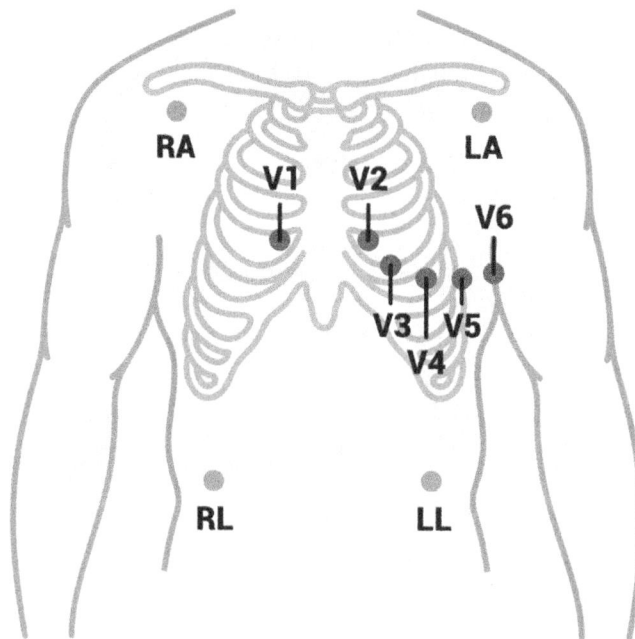

CAPTURING AN ECG

Steps for capturing a resting ECG include the following:

1. Introduce oneself and confirm the identity of the patient using two patient identifiers.
2. Explain the procedure, clarifying in layman's terms that the ECG will be capturing a picture of the heart rhythm that will involve no pain. Talk through the steps that will be taken, including describing the "stickers" (electrodes) that will be placed on the patient.
3. Turn on the ECG machine and fill in the required patient data, including name, age, sex, and indication for the ECG.
4. Attach the electrodes to the patient in the appropriate locations, ensuring to avoid bony prominences and dense fatty tissue/muscle. Shave the patient if necessary. Pat the patient's skin dry if perspiration is evident and use an alcohol pad if the patient's skin is oily. Attach the leads to the electrodes, paying attention to their labels: LA, LL, RA, RL and V1–V6.
5. Review the ECG preview screen to ensure all leads are properly placed and without artifact. Some ECG machines will alert for artifact. Remind the patient (and providers who are interacting with the patient) not to move or speak while the image is acquired.
6. Initiate capture. Wait patiently while the ECG machine acquires and prints the ECG. Tear the ECG report from the printer.
7. Review the ECG for artifact or malfunctioning leads.
8. Clean the ECG machine with the proper disinfectant based on the precautions required by the patient's condition. Remove the ECG and the ECG machine from the patient's room, and return to proper location.

ELEMENTS OF A COMPLETE ECG TRACING

The elements of a complete ECG tracing include:

- **Isoelectric line:** The baseline of the ECG during which there is no depolarization or repolarization occurring and the heart is at rest.
- **Wave:** A positive or negative deflection from the baseline, representing electrical activity of the heart, such as atrial depolarization (P wave) and ventricular repolarization (T wave). The U wave, present on some ECGs after the T wave, represents late ventricular repolarization.
- **Segment:** A part of the ECG tracing during which there is no electrical activity, such as the P-R segment and the S-T segment. Segments should be on or near the isoelectric line.
- **Interval:** A part of the ECG tracing that includes both a wave and a segment, such as the P-R interval and the Q-T interval.
- **Complex:** A group of waves that occur together, representing a single electrical event, such as the QRS complex, which represents ventricular depolarization.

ECG Acquisition

VERIFYING ECG SPEED AND GAIN SETTINGS

Speed is the rate at which the ECG paper moves through the print head—it is usually set at 25 millimeters per second (mm/s), although a healthcare provider may order that the speed be adjusted to 50 mm/s for greater clarity, such as with pediatric patients who have a more rapid pulse than adults. **Gain** refers to the vertical amplitude of a waveform. Gain is usually set at 10 mm/mV, and the calibration signal should produce a 10 mm deflection. If signals are small and difficult to read, then gain may be adjusted to 20 mm/mV to increase the size of the waveform, although it is not necessary to do so when increasing speed to 50 mm/s. Steps in the verification process may vary somewhat according to the manufacturer's guidelines but typically include:

- Access the settings menu.
- Determine if the settings are as prescribed, typically to standard values.
- Run a calibration test: Most current equipment has a built-in calibration function to verify settings.
- If the calibration signal does not match the expected values for the setting, adjust it accordingly.

MAINTAINING ECG EQUIPMENT

Note that the manufacturer's user manual should always be consulted regarding the **maintenance of ECG equipment** because procedures may vary. Maintenance of ECG equipment includes:

- **Paper loading:** Turn off the machine, unplugging it if necessary, to gain access to the print tray. Access the print tray and insert the paper roll or z-fold stack inside (depending on the type of machine) so that the printed/thermal side faces the print head. Align the paper with the feed mechanism and leave a section extending to the outside of the machine. Close the compartment.
- **Clip replacement:** Clips may need to be replaced if they are corroded, have poor grip or contact, have visible damage, have repeatedly poor transmission (e.g., "lead off" warning, inconsistent waveforms), and when there are persistent lead connection errors or increased artifacts. Determine the type of clip (e.g., snap, alligator, pinch) and order or request replacements. Remove the old clips and connect the new clips to the lead wires.
- **Necessary supplies:** ECG machine (properly calibrated), electrodes, electrode clips/adaptors, conductive gel, recording paper (appropriate for the ECG model), and skin preparation supplies (e.g., clipper, razor, alcohol wipes, abrasive tape/pads).

CLEANING AND STORAGE OF THE ECG MACHINE

Following the ECG, the technician must disinfect the ECG machine. The ECG machine is used across patient rooms; therefore, all bacteria must be removed prior to removing the ECG machine and using it on another patient. While wearing gloves, disinfect the machine using the proper disinfectant identified for this patient based on their level of isolation. Wipe down the entire machine, being sure to wipe each wire and lead. Remove gloves, wash hands, and exit the patient room with the ECG machine. Every unit should have a docking station for their ECG machine. It is the responsibility of the ECG technician to know where this docking station is located. Return the ECG machine to the docking station and plug it in to the power source to ensure power is available for the next ECG ordered. Apply a "clean" tag to the ECG machine to confirm that it has been properly disinfected after patient use.

PERMANENT RECORD OF ECG FOR PATIENT'S CHART

While **recording the ECG**, mark the leads on the top while changing the dial to different lead settings. To make a permanent record of a strip ECG, cut it to fit an 8.5" x 11" mounting card that fits in the chart. Examine the recording, and find one accurate representative example of each lead for the permanent record (I, II, III, AVR, AVL, AVF, V1, V2, V3, V4, V5, and V6). The example must not wander from the baseline, should contain any ectopic beats, and must contain a 1-milivolt standard deflection for comparison to the wave height. If there is a run of irregular beats, include it as a fold-over. Cut the example to fit the appropriate section of the mounting card. Peel back the cover over the adhesive, and press the cutting onto the card. Include a long rhythm strip from Lead II. Note if the patient is taking cardiac drugs, such as digoxin, or if he or she had difficulty breathing (dyspnea) or complained of chest pain during the recording.

ECG Acquisition

Skin Preparation and Patient Positioning

SKIN PREPARATION FOR ELECTRODE PLACEMENT

Steps to **preparing the skin for electrode placement** include:

- Asking about allergies or skin sensitivities to any products being used for the ECG
- Inspecting the skin for signs of sweat, oils, lotions, irritation, or excessive hair
- Identifying the location for electrodes. Note that underwire bras should be removed since they may cause artifacts, and front-closure bras often interfere with placement of V1 and V2 leads. Sports bras or wireless bras may be left on only if they do not interfere with the placement of the electrodes. Leads V4, V5, and V6 should be placed under the breast.
- Removing excess hair by shaving or clipping (electric clippers are preferred to razors) because hair may interfere with electrode contact
- Cleansing skin with alcohol pads, rubbing to remove any residue on the skin
- Abrading the skin with a gauze or abrasive pad, if necessary, for dry or thick skin
- Ensuring that the skin is completely dry before placing electrodes to ensure electrode adhesion
- Checking gel electrodes to ensure they are not dried out
- Applying electrodes as needed, depending on the number of leads, by pressing firmly and avoiding bony prominences, skin folds, and areas of skin irritation
- Running a test strip to ensure that a clear signal is received

PATIENT POSITIONING FOR SPECIAL POPULATIONS

Patient positioning considerations for special populations include the following:

- **Respiratory issues:** If unable to tolerate supine position, patients should be placed in semi-Fowler's (30–45°) to reduce respiratory distress. The head should be supported with pillows. The patient should be observed for use of accessory muscles, and the position should be modified as needed to reduce labored breathing. With a barrel chest, electrodes may need to be placed slightly lower than usual.
- **Amputees:** Patients can usually tolerate supine or semi-Fowler's position unless they have respiratory problems. Electrodes should be placed on the part of the body closest to the missing limb. For example, place electrodes above the hip or on the shoulder.
- **Late-term pregnancy:** Supine positioning may cause supine hypotension syndrome because of uterine compression of the vena cava; therefore, the patient should be placed in left lateral tilt (15–30°) or semi-Fowler's position. Electrode placement is essentially the same as for a nonpregnant patient except that, if the patient has peripheral edema or is in left lateral tilt position, the lower limb electrodes may need to be placed on the thigh or lower abdomen to improve the signal.

PATIENT POSITIONING FOR SPECIFIC CARDIAC TESTS

Patient positioning for specific cardiac tests includes:

- **Resting ECG**: The patient is placed in flat supine position unless modification is needed because of physical issues, such as pregnancy or respiratory distress.
- **Treadmill/cycle ergometer**: The patient is assisted onto the treadmill in a standing upright position or is assisted to sit on the cycle ergometer.
- **Holter monitor**: The patient is typically ambulatory during testing unless physically disabled.
- **Echocardiogram**: The patient is positioned in the left lateral decubitus position.
- **Single-photon emission computed tomography:** Most of the test is completed with the patient in supine position.
- **Nuclear stress test**: The patient is in supine position during imaging and upright during the stress testing phase.
- **Tilt-table test**: The patient is in supine position and then tilted upward to 60–80° to assess for orthostatic changes.
- **Electrophysiology study**: The patient is placed in supine position under moderate sedation. Electrodes are not placed on the skin because the heart is monitored through a catheter with an electrode tip.
- **BP monitoring**: The patient is typically seated with legs uncrossed.

ECG Acquisition

Electrode and Lead Application

AMBULATORY AND STATIONARY CARDIAC MONITORING

Ambulatory monitoring involves the following:

- Holter monitors: Worn for 24–48 hours, available in lead type or patch type.
- Event recorders: Worn for weeks to months. Records when activated.
- Implantable loop recorders: Implanted subcutaneously in the chest to monitor cardiac rhythms for up to 3 years.
- Wearable smart devices, such as the Apple Watch and KardiaMobile: Able to detect atrial fibrillation and other arrhythmias. Can transmit data to the physician.

Stationary monitoring involves the following:

- Bedside telemetry: This is partially stationary because the patient is confined to a limited space, such as a hospital unit. The patient wears electrodes connected to a transmitter to wirelessly transmit real-time cardiac data to a central monitoring station.
- Hardwired continuous ECG monitoring: Electrodes connect to a bedside monitor, so the patient is confined to the bed or must disconnect the leads in order to ambulate.

ELECTRODE PLACEMENT FOR AMBULATORY MONITORING

Electrode placement is dependent on the test:

- **Ambulatory monitoring (5-lead Holter):** A 5-lead configuration is typically used:
  - RA (white): Right upper chest, below the clavicle
  - LA (black): Left upper chest, below the clavicle
  - LL (red): Upper left abdomen
  - RL (green): Upper right abdomen
  - VI or C (brown): Fourth intercostal space, right of the sternum
- **Ambulatory monitoring (7-lead Holter):** A 7-lead (modified 12-lead) configuration is sometimes used with two additional electrodes:
  - V3 (orange): Midway between the fourth intercostal space left of the sternum (V2 position) and the fifth intercostal space, midclavicular line (V4 position)
  - V5 (purple): Left anterior axillary line, fifth intercostal space
- **Ambulatory monitoring (event):** A 3-lead configuration is typically used:
  - RA: Right chest, below the clavicle
  - LA: Left chest below the clavicle
  - LL: Lower left chest or upper abdomen

ELECTRODE PLACEMENT FOR STRESS TESTING AND TELEMETRY

Electrode placement for stress testing and telemetry is as follows.

Stress testing: The modified Mason-Likar system is used with the limb electrodes moved to the torso to reduce movement artifacts:

- RA (white): Right clavicle, midclavicular line
- LA (black): Left clavicle, midclavicular line
- RL (green): Right lower rib cage
- LL (red): Left lower rib cage
- V1 (brown/red): Fourth intercostal space, right of the sternum
- V2 (brown/yellow): Fourth intercostal space, left of the sternum
- V3 (brown/green): Midway between V2 and V4
- V4 (brown/blue): Fifth intercostal space, midclavicular line
- V5 (brown/orange): Fifth intercostal space, anterior axillary line
- V6 (brown/violet): Fifth intercostal space, midaxillary line

Telemetry: 3- or 5-lead placement is typically used:

- RA (white): Right upper chest, below the clavicle
- LA (black): Left upper chest, below the clavicle
- LL (red): Upper left abdomen
- RL (green): Upper right abdomen (for 5-lead)
- VI or C (brown): Fourth intercostal space, right of the sternum (for 5-lead)

ELECTRODE PLACEMENT FOR RIGHT-SIDED HEARTS AND POSTERIOR MONITORING

Electrode placement for right-sided heart monitoring and posterior monitoring is as follows:

- **Right-sided heart monitoring:** In the rare condition in which a patient's heart is located on the right side instead of the left (right-sided heart), the leads are placed in a mirror image to the lead placement for a standard left-sided heart. Leads are referred to as V1R, V2R, etc. The most critical lead for accurate monitoring is lead V4R, which must be placed in the 5th intercostal space on the right side, at the mid-clavicular line.
- **Posterior monitoring:** Used to assess posterior wall infarctions. Standard 12-lead electrode placement is used on the anterior chest for limb leads and V1 through V4, although V4 may be omitted. Leads V5 and V6 are typically omitted.

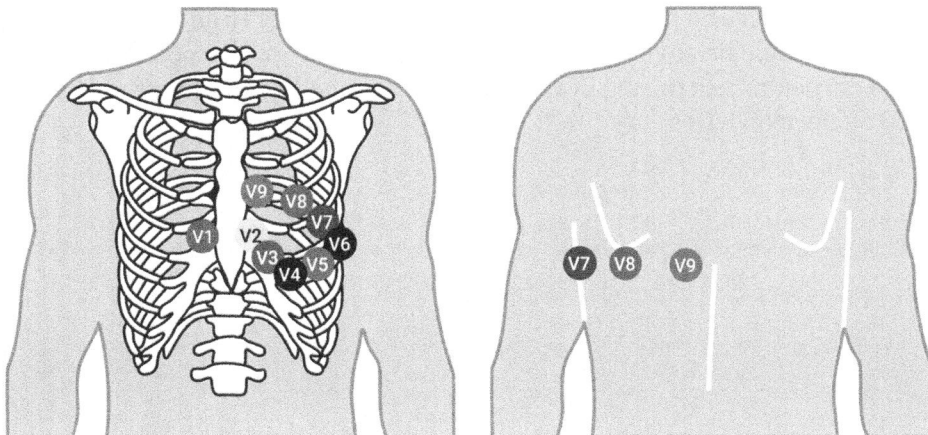

- **Posterior placement includes:**
  - ○ V7: Fifth intercostal space, posterior axillary line
  - ○ V8: Fifth intercostal space, posterior midscapular line
  - ○ V9: Fifth intercostal space, posterior left paraspinal line

ELECTRODE PLACEMENT FOR PEDIATRIC PATIENTS

Appropriately sized pediatric electrodes must be used in pediatric patients to prevent overlap. For very small infants, electrodes for leads V3–V6 may need to be placed slightly closer together. Limb electrodes are moved to the torso to reduce movement artifacts. Placement may be in relation to nipples for infants weighing less than 90 lb/41 kg because it may be too difficult to measure rib spaces:

- RA (white): Right clavicle or shoulder
- LA (black): Left clavicle or shoulder
- RL (green): Right lower torso
- LL (red): Left lower torso
- V1 (brown/red): Fourth intercostal space or nipple line, right of the sternum, a half inch from the midline
- V2 (brown/yellow): Fourth intercostal space or nipple line, left of the sternum, a half inch from the midline
- V3 (brown/green): Midway between V2 and V4
- V4 (brown/blue): Fifth intercostal space or below the nipple line at the midclavicular line, left side
- V5 (brown/orange): Fifth intercostal space, anterior axillary line, left side
- V6 (brown/violet): Fifth intercostal space, midaxillary line

ELECTRODE PLACEMENT FOR SPECIAL CONDITIONS

Capturing an ECG on a patient with special conditions requires the following considerations:

- **Amputee**: If the patient has an amputated limb, or a limb is not accessible for an electrode due to a dressing or wound, the priority is that the ECG leads are placed symmetrically on the body. For instance, if the right wrist of a patient is amputated, place the RA and LA electrodes on the soft tissue below the shoulder joint.
- **Pacemaker**: If a patient has a pacemaker, be sure not to place the electrode directly atop the pacemaker to avoid interference with the ECG reading. Place the electrode 3–5 inches from the pacemaker and place the RA electrode symmetrically on the other side of the body.
- **Piercings**: It should be advised that patient's remove all jewelry possible. Body piercings present a particular risk during ECG's and may be ripped out unintentionally after being snagged on the lead wires.

ECG Acquisition

ARTIFACTS ON THE ECG TRACING

The two most common **causes of artifact** on the ECG tracing are easily preventable:

- **Loose leads**: Electrodes may not have sufficient adhesion to the body, due to body hair, perspiration or oil on the skin, or lead location. To avoid this problem, quickly shave heavy body hair and wipe the skin of any perspiration or dampness. Use alcohol pads to effectively remove oil from the skin and allow the alcohol to dry. Select flat locations for electrode placement to prevent bending and folding of the electrode.
- **Patient movement**: Patient movement, such as shivering, coughing, or speaking, can cause a wandering baseline on the ECG reading. To avoid this, communicate with the patient prior to initiating the ECG reading, asking them to keep still. Also notify any of the health care members that may be working on the patient, so that they can step back and refrain from moving the patient during ECG capture. Make sure the patient is warm to prevent shivering.

TYPES OF ECG ARTIFACTS

Artifact	Description	Solution
Wandering baseline	The baseline drifts up and down, typically caused by poor preparation of skin, improper electrode placement, or very deep breathing during recording.	Clean the skin thoroughly and apply the electrodes properly, shaving or clipping the hair as necessary for adhesion. Make sure that the gel on the electrodes is fresh. Encourage the patient to relax and breathe evenly.
Somatic tremor	Rapid, irregular fluctuations from the baseline because of muscle activity resulting from tremors (such as with Parkinson's disease), shivering, tension, or movement during recording.	Keep the patient warm, encourage relaxation, position the electrodes on the upper chest and trunk instead of on the arms and legs if necessary.
AC/60-cycle interference	Uniform, regular, equally spaced, small vertical spikes, usually affecting all leads resulting from electrical interference from nearby power cords, electrical devices, an improperly grounded ECG machine, loose electrodes, cell phones, or fluorescent lights.	Prepare the skin properly, check electrodes and wire positioning, prevent leads from touching each other, keep the ECG machine at least 3 feet from other power sources, turn off nearby electrical devices if possible, turn off fluorescent lights, ensure that the ECG machine is properly grounded, and use a machine with a notch filter to reduce interference.

MONITORING PATIENTS DURING STRESS TESTING

The role of the ECG technician in monitoring patients during stress testing includes:

- Explaining the procedure to the patient and helping the patient to prepare
- Calculating the target heart rate, using the appropriate formula
- Obtaining a baseline ECG with the patient in supine position
- Assisting the patient to a sitting and then a standing position
- Applying a BP cuff and pulse oximeter and taking baseline vital signs and oxygen saturation
- Setting the BP cuff for automatic readings, usually every 2 minutes
- Assisting the patient onto the treadmill or cycle ergometer
- Monitoring continuously during the stress test for heart rate, BP, oxygen saturation, and adverse symptoms
- Repeating ECGs according to facility guidelines, typically every 2 to 3 minutes
- Assisting the healthcare provider as needed and alerting the healthcare provider to adverse symptoms or changes in vital signs or oxygen saturation
- Assisting the patient to step down from the treadmill or cycle ergometer and ensuring that the patient is stable
- Continuing with monitoring until the patient's vital signs and oxygen saturation return to baseline, usually within 15 minutes
- Disconnecting leads and electrodes and discarding the electrodes
- Documenting and uploading/transmitting the ECG to the patient's electronic health record

EMERGENCIES THAT MAY OCCUR

Emergencies that may occur during stress testing:

- **Changes in cardiac status:** The heart rate usually increases about 10 beats per minute per level of exertion. Tachycardia beyond the maximum predicted heart rate, bradycardia (<60), hypotension, and hypertension indicate a cardiac emergency. ECG changes that signal an emergency include ST elevation or depression (common in myocardial infarction) and lethal dysrhythmias (e.g., ventricular tachycardia, ventricular fibrillation, third-degree heart block, agonal rhythm, pulseless electrical activity, and asystole).
- **Shortness of breath:** A normal increase in the patient's respiratory rate may be up to 30–40 during peak exercise, but the patient should not feel acutely short of breath or appear cyanotic.
- **Chest pain/pressure:** Pain or pressure in the chest with or without radiating pain to the neck and left arm or back with diaphoresis indicates an emergency.
- **Changes in mental status/dizziness:** Indicate that the blood supply to the brain is inadequate (e.g., hypotension, arrhythmias, or impending stroke).
- **Increased weakness or instability**.

The emergency response includes immediately stopping the test, assisting the patient into a sitting position (or lying if unconscious), calling for help according to the facility protocol, performing an ECG, and checking patient vital signs. If the patient is in cardiac arrest, then start cardiopulmonary resuscitation.

ECG Analysis and Interpretation

Calculations

FORMULAS FOR CALCULATING MAXIMUM HEART RATE
FOX AND HASKELL, GELLISH, GULATI, AND TANAKA

The MHR is the highest heart rate that the body can achieve at maximum effort. It tends to decrease with age. Formulas for finding the **MHR** with an example of a 56-year-old (results are rounded) are as follows:

Model	MHR Formula	Example	Note
Fox and Haskell	220 – age	220 – 56 = 164	Less accurate for older adults or athletes; good for general fitness
Gellish	207 – (0.7 × age)	207 – 39.2 = 168	More accurate for athletes
Gulati	206 – (0.88 × age)	206 – 49.28 = 157	More accurate for females
Tanaka	208 – (0.7 × age)	208 – 39.2 = 169	More accurate for older adults

PERCENTAGE METHOD AND KARVONEN/HEART RATE RESERVE (HRR) METHOD

Formulas for finding the **target heart rate (THR)** use the MHR. For these examples, the Fox and Haskell model is used to determine the MHR with a patient aged 56 and MHR of 164 (the results are rounded):

Method	Formula	Additional Info	Example
Percentage	MHR × exercise intensity percentage = THR	Exercise intensity: 50–60% light 60–70% moderate 70–85% vigorous 85–100% maximal	For light intensity: 164 × 0.60 = 98 THR
Karvonen/ heart rate reserve (HRR)	Three steps: 1. MHR – resting heart rate (RHR) = HRR 2. HRR × exercise intensity percentage 3. Add the RHR	RHR = first AM heart rate	164 – 76 (RHR) = 88 (HRR) 88 × 0.60 = 52.8 52.8 + 76 = 129 (THR)

R-R INTERVAL AND SEQUENCING METHODS

Methods used to quickly estimate heart rate include the following:

- The **6-second method**: Every 30 large boxes/150 small boxes equal 6 seconds (usually marked by hashmarks at the top of the tracing): Count the number of QRS complexes in a 6-second strip and multiply by 10. This method is often used to estimate when the heart rate is regular, but it may also be used when it is regularly irregular (such as in atrial fibrillation).
- **R-R interval method:** Assesses the heart rate between R waves. The heart rate must be regular: Count the number of small boxes between two consecutive R waves and divide 1,500 (i.e., the number of small boxes that equal 1 minute) by this number.
- **Sequencing method:** Requires memorization of the sequence 300, 150, 75, 60, 50, 43, 37. This can be used to rapidly estimate the heart rate using the R-R interval with a regular heart rate: since there are 17 small squares, a little less than half the distance between 15 and 20 small squares, the heart rate is between 75 and 100 beats per minute: 88.

Small squares	Large squares	Bpm
5	1	300
10	2	150
15	3	100
20	4	75
25	5	60
30	6	50
35	7	43
40	8	37

UNITS OF MEASUREMENT USED FOR ECG GRAPH PAPER

The horizontal (x) axis represents time. The typical speed for recording an ECG is 25 mm per second (mm/s), although, for some cases, such as pediatric patients, a rate of 50 mm/s may be used to allow the waveform to expand to provide better detail. Each large block is 5 mm in width, so at the usual speed of 25 mm/s, 1 large block represents 0.20 seconds. Each small block is 1 mm in width, or 0.04 seconds at 25 mm/s. Equivalently, 5 large blocks or 25 small blocks equal 1 second, and 300 large blocks or 1,500 small blocks equal 1 minute.

The vertical (y) axis measures the amplitude/voltage. ECG machines are typically calibrated so that 1 mV produces a 10 mm deflection (2 large squares). The height of each small square then represents 0.1 mV, and the height of each large square represents 0.5 mV.

If using the 50 mm/s rate, interval adjustments are needed because the waveform will be twice as wide:

Measure	25 mm/s	50 mm/s
Small square	0.04 second	0.02 second
Large square	0.20 second	0.10 second

Interpretation

ATRIAL AND VENTRICULAR ABNORMALITIES

PREMATURE VENTRICULAR CONTRACTIONS

Premature ventricular contractions (PVCs) are those in which the impulse begins in the ventricles and conducts through them prior to the next sinus impulse. PVCs usually cause no morbidity unless there is underlying cardiac disease or an acute MI. PVCs are characterized by an irregular heartbeat, QRS that is ≥0.12 seconds and oddly shaped. PVCs are often not treated in otherwise healthy people. PVCs may be precipitated by electrolyte imbalances, caffeine, nicotine, or alcohol. The nurse should be notified if PVCs become frequent and/or the patient is complaining of discomfort.

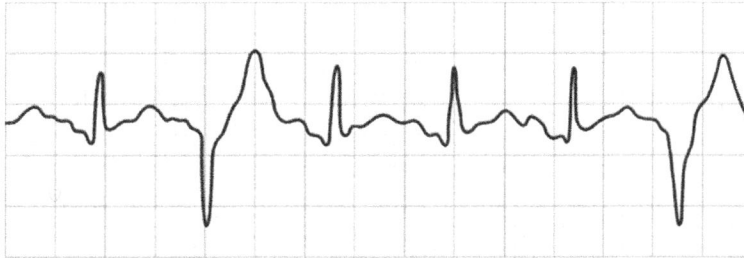

PREMATURE ATRIAL CONTRACTIONS

Premature atrial contraction (PAC) is essentially an extra beat precipitated by an electrical impulse to the atrium before the sinus node impulse. The extra beat may be caused by alcohol, caffeine, nicotine, hypervolemia, hypokalemia, hypermetabolic conditions, atrial ischemia, or infarction. Characteristics include an irregular pulse because of extra P waves, the shape and duration of QRS is usually normal (0.04–0.11 seconds) but may be abnormal, PR interval remains between 0.12–0.20, and P:QRS ratio is 1:1. Rhythm is irregular with varying P-P and R-R intervals.

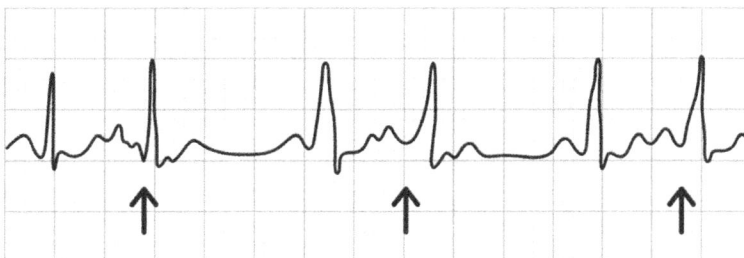

PACs can occur in an essentially healthy heart and are not usually cause for concern unless they are frequent (>6 per hr) and cause severe palpitations. In that case, the nurse should be notified.

ECG Analysis and Interpretation

IRREGULAR RHYTHMS

SINUS BRADYCARDIA

Sinus bradycardia (SB) is caused by a decreased rate of impulse from sinus node. The pulse and ECG usually appear normal except for a slower rate.

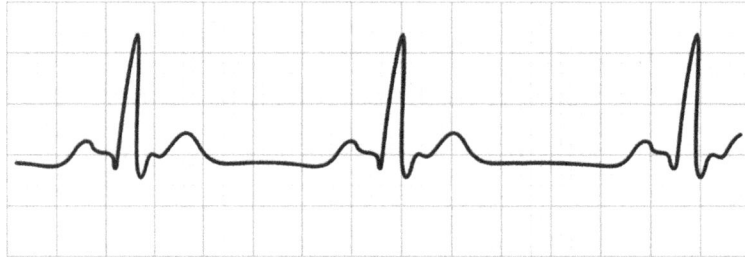

SB is characterized by a regular pulse <50–60 bpm with P waves in front of QRS, which are usually normal in shape and duration. PR interval is 0.12–0.20 seconds, QRS interval is 0.04–0.11 seconds, and P:QRS ratio of 1:1. Some individuals may naturally have a slower heart rate. If the patient is complaining of dizziness or has mental status changes, notify the nurse immediately.

SINUS TACHYCARDIA

Sinus tachycardia (ST) occurs when the sinus node impulse increases in frequency. ST is characterized by a regular pulse >100 with P waves before QRS but sometimes part of the preceding T wave. QRS is usually of normal shape and duration (0.04–0.11 seconds) but may have consistent irregularity. PR interval is 0.12–0.20 seconds and P:QRS ratio of 1:1.

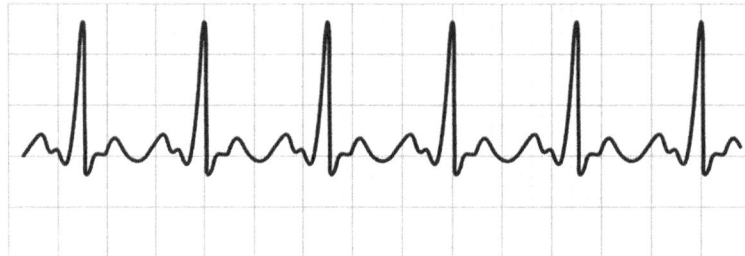

Sinus tachycardia can be caused by a variety of factors, to include pain, anxiety, dehydration, or decreased blood pressure.

ATRIAL FIBRILLATION

Atrial fibrillation (A-fib) is rapid, disorganized atrial beats that are ineffective in emptying the atria, so that blood pools in the chambers. This can lead to thrombus formation and emboli. A-fib is caused by coronary artery disease, valvular disease, pulmonary disease, heavy alcohol ingestion, infection, and cardiac surgery; however, it can also be idiopathic. A-fib is characterized by a very irregular pulse with atrial rate of 300–600 and ventricular rate of 120–200, shape and duration (0.04–0.11 seconds) of QRS is usually normal. Fibrillatory (F) waves are seen instead of P waves. The PR interval cannot be measured and the P:QRS ratio is highly variable.

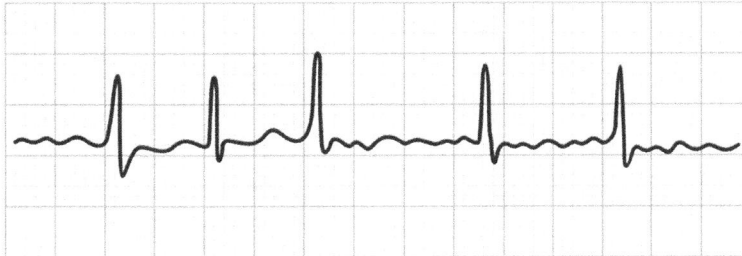

ATRIAL FLUTTER

Atrial flutter (AF) occurs when the atrial rate is faster, usually 250–400 beats per minute, than the AV node conduction rate so not all of the beats are conducted into the ventricles. AF is caused by the same conditions that cause A-fib: coronary artery disease, valvular disease, pulmonary disease, heavy alcohol ingestion, and cardiac surgery. AF is characterized by atrial rates of 250–400 with ventricular rates of 75–150, with ventricular rate usually being regular. P waves are saw-toothed (referred to as F waves), QRS shape and duration (0.04–0.11 seconds) are usually normal, PR interval may be hard to calculate because of F waves, and the P:QRS ratio is 2:1 to 4:1. Symptoms include chest pain, dyspnea, and hypotension.

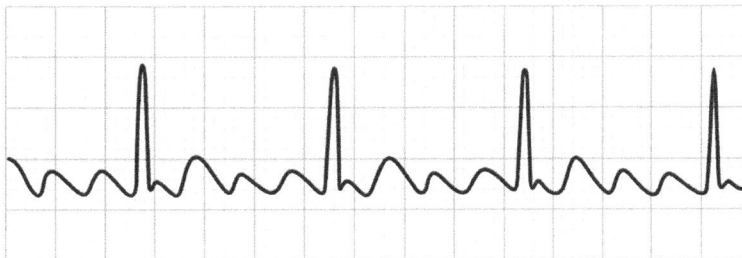

ECG Analysis and Interpretation

VENTRICULAR TACHYCARDIA

Ventricular tachycardia (VT) is greater than 3 PVCs in a row with a ventricular rate of 100–200 beats per minute. This is a dangerous rhythm if left untreated, and the nurse should be notified immediately. The rapid rate of contractions makes VT dangerous as the ineffective beats may render the person unconscious with no palpable pulse. A detectable rate is usually regular and the QRS complex is ≥0.12 seconds and is usually abnormally shaped. The P wave may be undetectable with an irregular PR interval if P wave is present. The P:QRS ratio is often difficult to ascertain because of the absence of P waves.

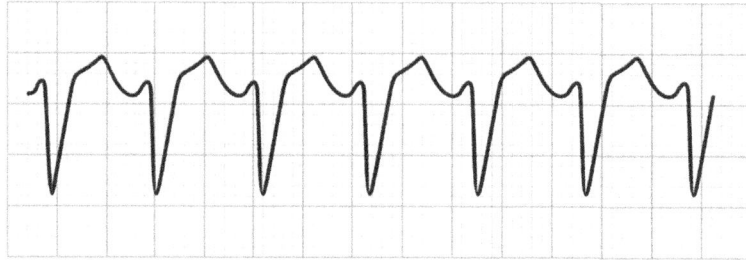

VENTRICULAR FIBRILLATION

Ventricular fibrillation (VF) is a rapid, very irregular ventricular rate >300 beats per minute with no atrial activity observable on the ECG, caused by disorganized electrical activity in the ventricles. The QRS complex is not recognizable as ECG shows irregular undulations. The causes are the same as for ventricular tachycardia and asystole. VF is accompanied by lack of palpable pulse, audible pulse, and respirations and is immediately life threatening without defibrillation. This is a medical emergency and a code blue should be called if witnessed with no immediate help available.

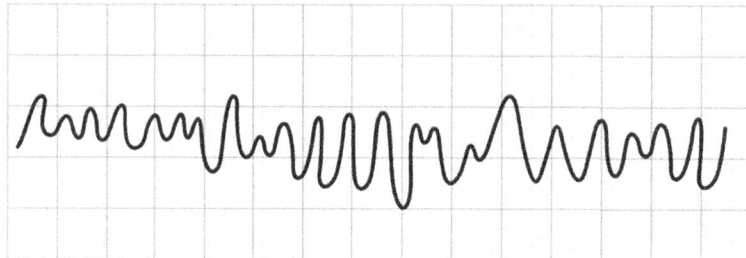

ASYSTOLE

Ventricular asystole is the absence of audible heartbeat, palpable pulse, and respirations, a condition often referred to as "cardiac arrest." While the ECG may show some P waves initially, the QRS complex is absent although there may be an occasional QRS "escape beat" (agonal rhythm). If this is seen on the monitor, first observe the patient in case the leads have been detached. If the patient is unresponsive, cardiopulmonary resuscitation is required with intubation for ventilation and establishment of an intravenous line for fluids. Without immediate treatment, the patient will suffer from severe hypoxia and brain death within minutes. Even with immediate treatment, the prognosis is poor and ventricular asystole is often a sign of impending death.

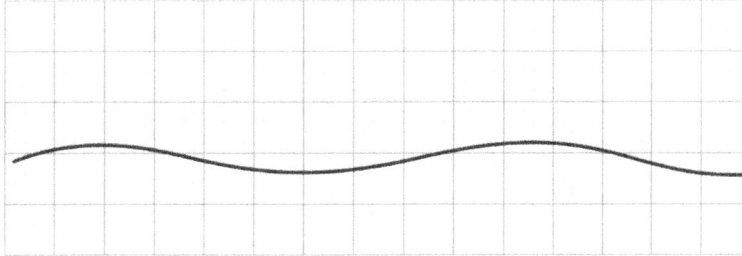

HEART BLOCKS

FIRST-DEGREE AV BLOCK

Heart blocks are categorized by severity in degrees. Any heart block identified on ECG requires nurse notification, particularly if it is new and/or the patient is symptomatic. While some heart blocks are benign, others can be life-threatening if not immediately treated.

First-degree AV block occurs when the atrial impulses are conducted through the AV node to the ventricles at a rate that is slower than normal. While the P and QRS are usually normal, the PR interval is >0.20 seconds, and the P:QRS ratio is 1:1. A narrow QRS complex indicates a conduction abnormality only in the AV node, but a widened QRS indicates associated damage to the bundle branches as well.

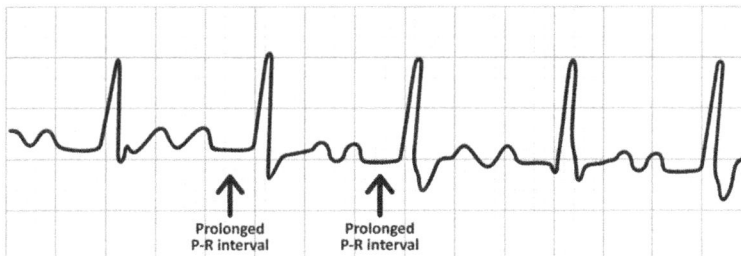

SECOND-DEGREE AV BLOCK

Second-degree AV block occurs when some of the atrial beats are blocked. Second-degree AV block is further subdivided according to the patterns of block.

ECG Analysis and Interpretation

63

TYPE I

Mobitz type I block (Wenckebach) occurs when each atrial impulse in a group of beats is conducted at a lengthened interval until one fails to conduct (the PR interval progressively increases), so there are more P waves than QRS complexes, but the QRS complex is usually of normal shape and duration. The sinus node functions at a regular rate, so the P-P interval is regular, but the R-R interval usually shortens with each impulse. The P:QRS ratio varies, such as 3:2, 4:3, 5:4. This type of block by itself usually does not cause significant morbidity unless associated with an inferior wall myocardial infarction.

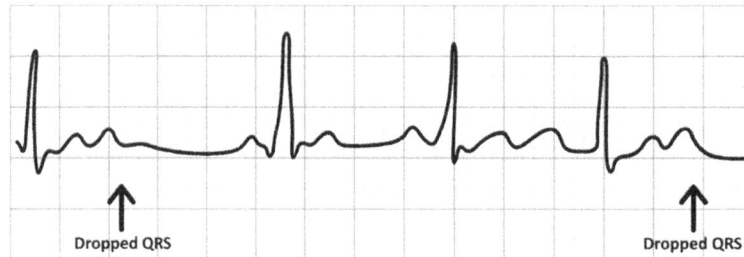

TYPE II

In Mobitz type II, only some of the atrial impulses are conducted unpredictably through the AV node to the ventricles, and the block always occurs below the AV node in the bundle of His, the bundle branches, or the Purkinje fibers. The PR intervals are the same if impulses are conducted, and the QRS complex is usually widened. The P:QRS ratio varies 2:1, 3:1, and 4:1. Type II block is more dangerous than Type I because it may progress to complete AV block and may produce Stokes-Adams syncope. Additionally, if the block is at the Purkinje fibers, there is no escape impulse. Usually, a transcutaneous cardiac pacemaker and defibrillator should be at the patient's bedside. **Symptoms** may include chest pain if the heart block is precipitated by myocarditis or myocardial ischemia.

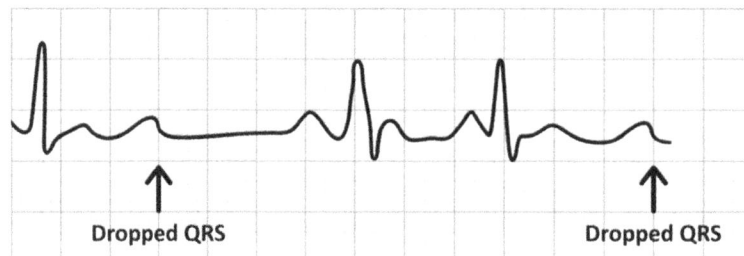

THIRD-DEGREE AV BLOCK

With third-degree AV block, there are more P waves than QRS complexes, with no clear relationship between them. The atrial rate is 2–3 times the pulse rate, so the PR interval is irregular. If the SA node malfunctions, the AV node fires at a lower rate, and if the AV node malfunctions, the pacemaker site in the ventricles takes over at a bradycardic rate; thus, with complete AV block, the heart still contracts, but often ineffectually. With this type of block, the atrial P (sinus rhythm or atrial fibrillation) and the ventricular QRS (ventricular escape rhythm) are stimulated by different impulses, so there is AV dissociation.

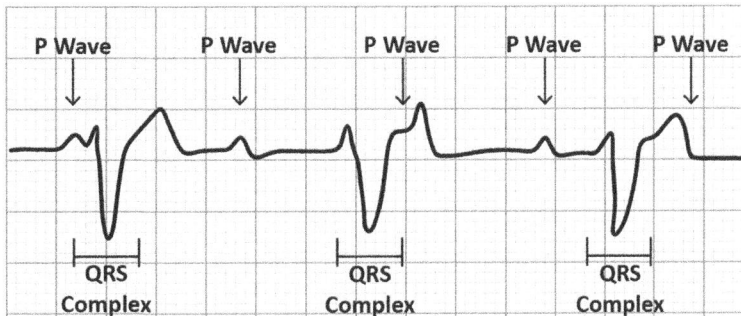

The heart may compensate at rest but can't keep pace with exertion. The resultant bradycardia may cause congestive heart failure, fainting, or even sudden death, and usually conduction abnormalities slowly worsen. Symptoms include dyspnea, chest pain, and hypotension, which are treated with IV atropine. Transcutaneous pacing may be needed. Complete persistent AV block normally requires implanted pacemakers, usually dual chamber.

> **Review Video: AV Heart Blocks**
> Visit mometrix.com/academy and enter code: 487004

ECG Analysis and Interpretation

BUNDLE BRANCH BLOCKS

A **right bundle branch block (RBBB)** occurs when conduction is blocked in the right bundle branch that carries impulses from the Bundle of His to the right ventricle. The impulse travels through the left ventricle instead, and then reaches the right ventricle, but this causes a slight delay in contraction of the right ventricle. A RBBB is characterized by normal P waves (as the right atrium still contracts appropriately), but the QRS complex is widened and notched (referred to as an "RSR pattern" that resembles the letter "M") in lead V1, which is a reflection of the asynchronous ventricular contraction. The PR interval is normal or prolonged, and the QRS interval is > 0.12 seconds. P:QRS ratio remains 1:1 with regular rhythms.

A **left bundle branch block (LBBB)** occurs when there is a delay in conduction between the left atrium and left ventricle. It is also characterized by normal or inverted P waves, but the QRS complex may be widened with a deep S wave and an interval of >0.12 seconds (in lead V1) that resembles a "W." The PR interval may be normal or prolonged. The P:QRS ratio is 1:1 and the rhythm is regular.

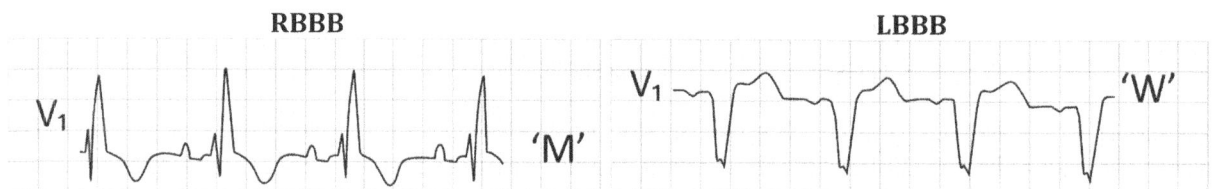

PACED RHYTHMS

Some patients requiring an ECG may have a pacemaker in place. This appears on ECG and the technician should be familiar with what to expect for these patients. Pacemaker capture occurs when an artificial stimulus (the pulse generator) depolarizes the heart, indicated by a pacer spike followed by the QRS complex. The pacer spike will appear as a straight line and should immediately be followed by a normal-appearing QRS complex.

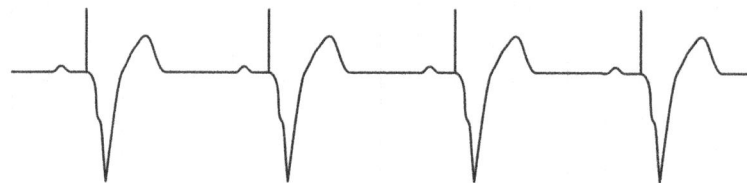

66

COMMON ECG PROBLEMS

Pacemakers may not be functioning properly, and the ECG technician must notify the nurse when evidence of pacemaker dysfunction is noted.

UNDERSENSING

The sensitivity is too low to detect cardiac depolarizations, and triggers unneeded contractions, competing with the patient's native rhythm. This may be related to the dislodging of the lead, incorrect positioning of the lead, or a low-amplitude cardiac signal.

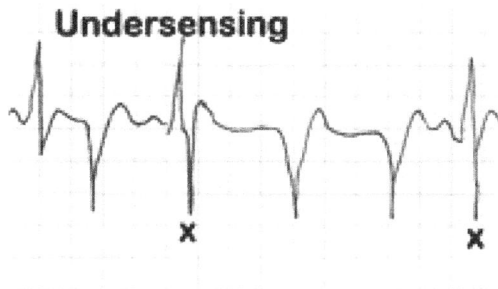

Undersensing

OVERSENSING

The sensitivity is too high and misinterprets artifacts (such as muscle contractions) and non-depolarization events as contractions and fails to trigger, resulting in decreased cardiac output because of the interruption in contractions. This may result from damage or disconnection of the lead.

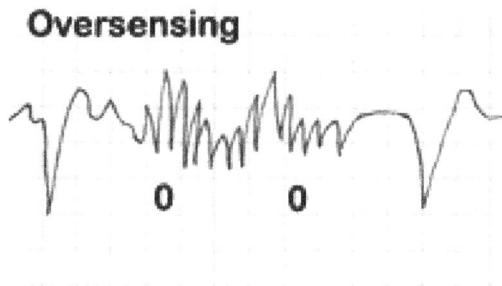

Oversensing

NONCAPTURE

The pacemaker does not trigger contractions. This may be related to settings, lead disconnection, low battery, or metabolic changes.

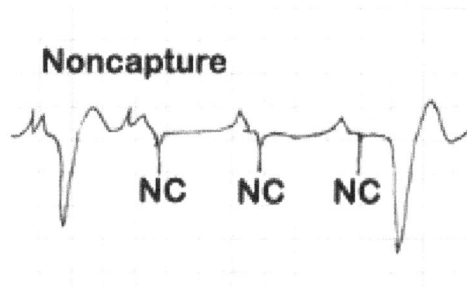

Noncapture

ECG Analysis and Interpretation

EKG Tech Practice Test #1

Want to take this practice test in an online interactive format?
Check out the online resources page, which includes interactive practice
questions and much more: **mometrix.com/resources719/nhaekgtech**

1. A patient with a history of atrial fibrillation and a family history of sudden cardiac death before age 45 has the following EKG tracing with a coved elevated ST segment and a negative T wave. This is referred to as:

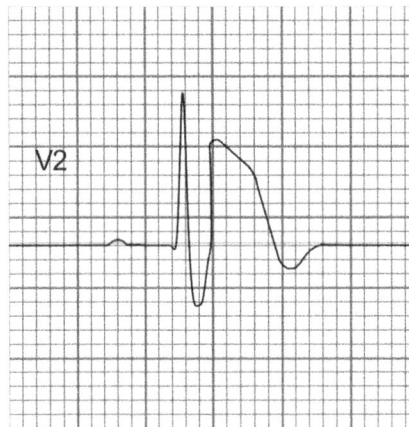

a. Epsilon wave
b. De Winter's sign
c. Brugada sign
d. Spiked helmet sign

2. When preparing to perform an EKG exam, an appropriate method of verifying the patient's identification is to:

a. Check the patient's armband.
b. Ask "What is your name and birthdate?"
c. Ask "Are you Alice Smith?"
d. Ask "Can you give me your identification?"

68

3. The following EKG tracing is an example of:

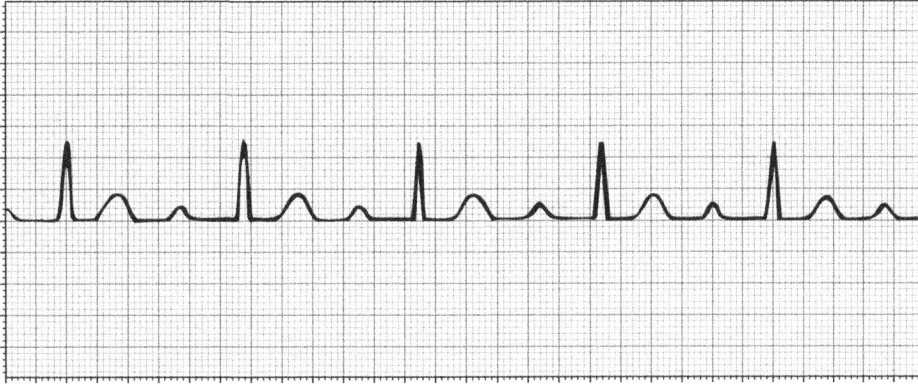

a. Sinus bradycardia
b. First-degree heart block
c. Left bundle branch block
d. Second-degree AV block

4. A dysrhythmia characterized by a regular heart rate of 150–250 bpm with abnormally shaped P waves (that may be hidden in the preceding T waves) but with a normal PR interval and normal QRS complex is:

a. Sinus tachycardia
b. Paroxysmal SVT
c. Junctional dysrhythmia
d. Atrial flutter

5. When interpreting an EKG tracing, if waves represent the same electrical event but are different in appearance, this is referred to as:

a. Aberrant
b. Biphasic
c. Monomorphic
d. Polymorphic

6. Which type of event recorder may be most indicated for a patient who has episodic ventricular tachycardia (VT) but is generally unaware of the symptoms?

a. Looping memory recorder
b. Postevent recorder
c. Autotriggered event monitor
d. Implantable loop recorder

7. Classic symptoms of pain related to angina are most often experienced in what three locations? (Select the three [3] correct answers.)

a. Chest
b. Right hand
c. Jaw
d. Abdomen
e. Left arm

8. This EKG tracing is indicative of:

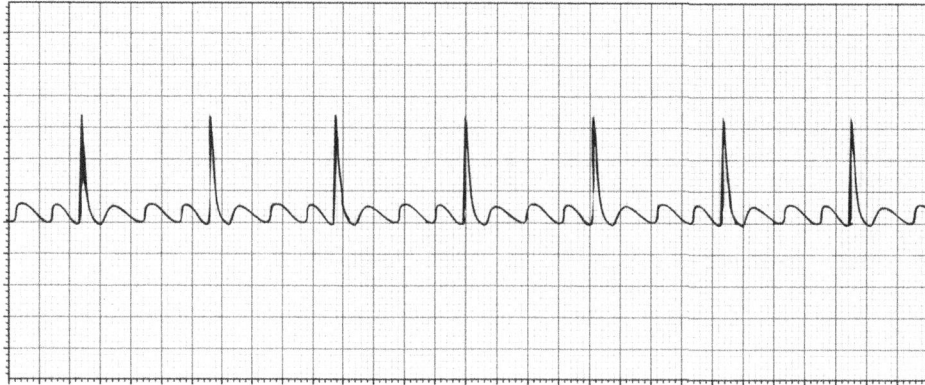

a. Atrial flutter
b. VT
c. Ventricular fibrillation
d. Atrial fibrillation

9. Leads aVR, aVL, and aVF use the same three electrodes as leads:

a. I, II, and III
b. V1, V2, and V3
c. II, III, and V
d. V4, V5, and V6

10. Which of the following is an open-ended question?

a. How did that make you feel?
b. Are you hungry?
c. Do you have any visual problems?
d. Are you a nurse?

11. What does this EKG tracing illustrate?

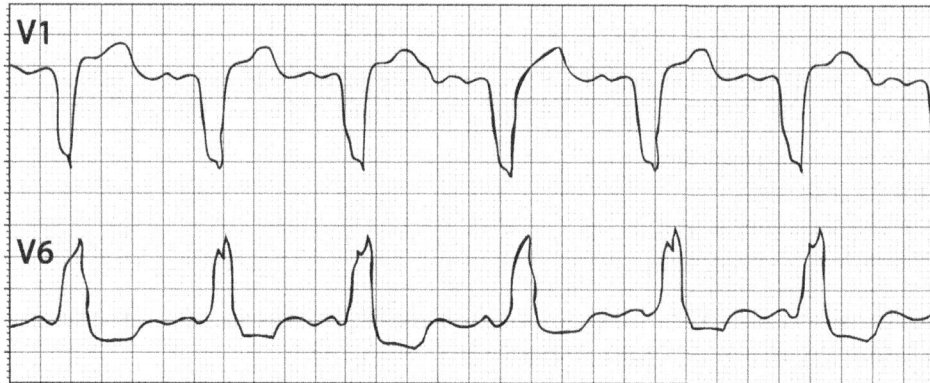

a. Normal sinus rhythm
b. Left bundle branch block
c. Right bundle branch block
d. Left ventricular hypertrophy

70

12. If a patient is to have a nuclear stress test, how many EKGs are typically done at the completion of the exercise portion of the test?

    a. Two
    b. Three
    c. Four
    d. Five

13. hat is the duration of the QRS complex on this EKG strip?

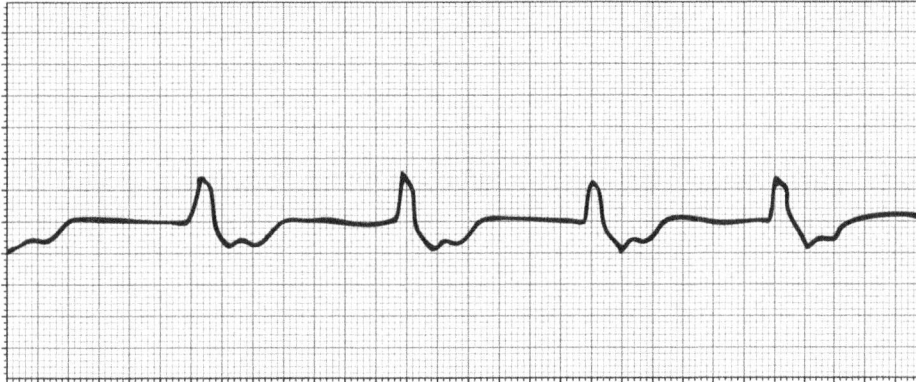

    a. 0.12 sec
    b. 0.14 sec
    c. 0.18 sec
    d. 0.22 sec

14. What is the duration of a normal QRS complex?

    a. 0.06–0.10 sec
    b. 0.12–0.20 sec
    c. 0.24–0.30 sec
    d. 0.36–0.44 sec

15. Which of the following is not a HIPAA violation?

    a. Having computer screens face into the main lobby.
    b. Disclosing a patient's medical information without consent.
    c. Discussing a patient's diagnosis in the waiting room.
    d. Sending a patient's records to their primary care doctor's office.

16. Which of the following statements belongs in the chief complaint section of a progress note?

    a. Abdominal pain for five days.
    b. Employed as a lawyer.
    c. Tylenol helping to alleviate pain.
    d. History of alcohol abuse.

17. A patient with osteoarthritis complains of pain in the knees during an exercise stress test when the incline increases. The best solution is likely to:

    a. Slow the speed.
    b. Modify the incline.
    c. Stop the test.
    d. Encourage the patient to continue.

18. An adult with a pulse rate of 70 beats per minute has:

    a. A normal pulse rate
    b. Bradycardia
    c. Tachycardia
    d. Arrhythmia

19. What artery is most commonly used when taking blood pressure?

    a. Femoral.
    b. Brachial.
    c. Subclavian.
    d. Jugular.

20. During an exercise stress test, an older patient complains of feeling nauseated and slightly dizzy. The patient appears pale, and his skin is clammy. The EKG technician should immediately:

    a. Call for help.
    b. Slow the speed of the exercise test.
    c. Ask the patient if he wants to stop the test.
    d. Assist the patient to sit.

21. When speaking to someone whose native language is not English, which of the following would not be helpful in communication with the patient?

    a. Having a translator present.
    b. Speaking slowly.
    c. Writing the instructions.
    d. Using hand gestures.

22. The slurred upstroke of the QRS complex is referred to as a(n):

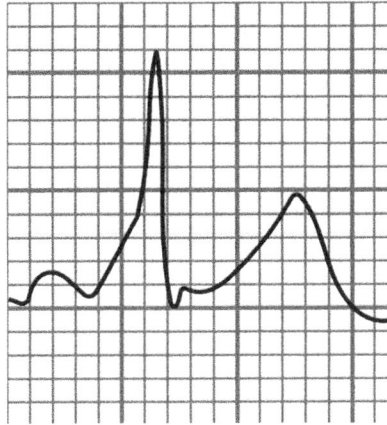

    a. De Winter's sign
    b. Spodick's sign
    c. Epsilon wave
    d. Delta wave

23. Which of the following would NOT be included in a living will?

    a. Whether a patient would like cardiopulmonary resuscitation (CPR) if cardiac arrest occurs
    b. If a patient would like to be kept alive with life-prolonging equipment
    c. If a patient does not want to have tube feeding
    d. How a person's assets should be distributed

24. What type of heart block does the following EKG tracing demonstrate?

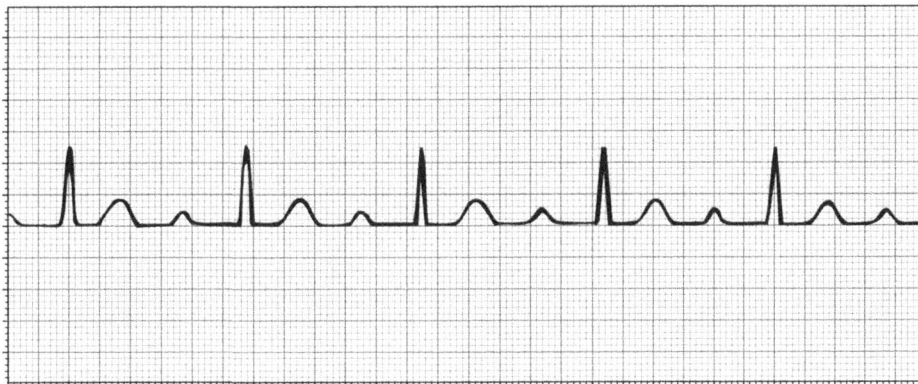

    a. First-degree AV block
    b. Second-degree AV block (Mobitz I)
    c. Second-degree AV block (Mobitz II)
    d. Left bundle branch block

25. Which one of the following leads aligns best with the natural depolarization of the heart?

    a. Lead I
    b. Lead II
    c. Lead III
    d. Lead V4

EKG Tech Practice Test #1

26. What layer of the skin contains blood vessels, nerve endings, and glands?

   a. Epidermis
   b. Dermis
   c. Hypodermis
   d. Integumentary

27. If performing an EKG exam on a child, it is most important to:

   a. Conduct the EKG exam quickly.
   b. Tell the child not to worry.
   c. Reassure the child that the EKG does not hurt.
   d. Distract the child by chatting during the EKG.

28. During an exercise stress test, the EKG technician notes that the patient frequently grimaces. The EKG technician should:

   a. Ask if the patient is having discomfort.
   b. Call for help.
   c. Stop the test.
   d. Take note of the frequency.

29. The following pattern on an EKG tracing is characteristic of:

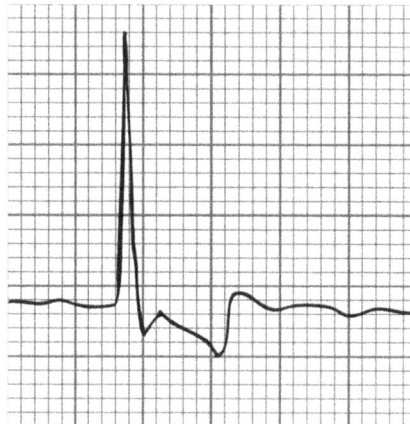

   a. Digoxin therapy
   b. Hypokalemia
   c. Ischemia
   d. Myocardial infarction

30. The rhythm for the following EKG tracing is best described as:

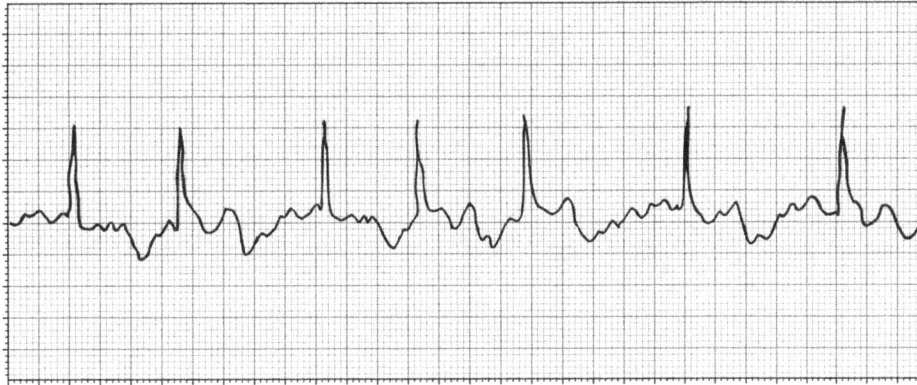

a. Atrial flutter
b. Atrial fibrillation
c. Premature atrial contractions
d. Ventricular fibrillation

31. The following EKG tracing is characteristic of which electrolyte imbalance?

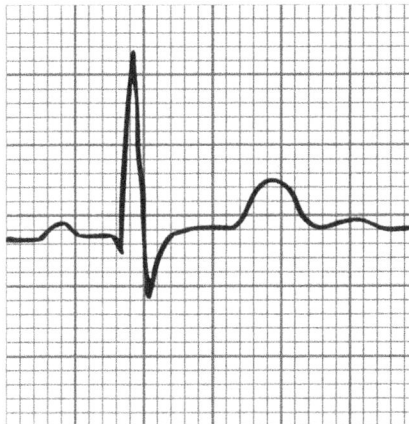

a. Hyperkalemia
b. Hypokalemia
c. Hypocalcemia
d. Hypomagnesemia

32. If the EKG technician notes the following EKG pattern, the first step is to:

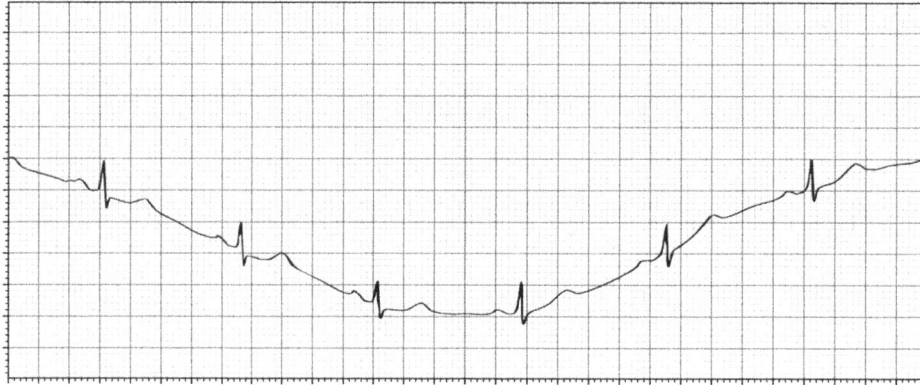

    a. Ask the patient to stay still and breathe normally.
    b. Check the EKG machine settings.
    c. Check the electrode placement.
    d. Support the lead wires.

33. The EKG technician needs to perform an EKG exam on a neonate who is crying and moving about. What is the best initial solution?

    a. Wait until the infant calms.
    b. Document the inability to perform the EKG.
    c. Ask if there are comfort measures available.
    d. Ask a parent to hold the infant during the EKG.

34. What is the approximate duration of the P-R interval on the following EKG tracing?

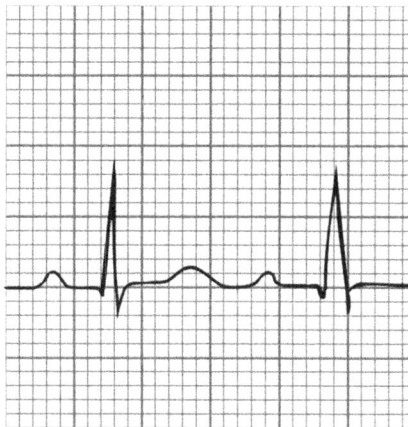

    a. 0.24 sec
    b. 0.20 sec
    c. 0.16 sec
    d. 0.12 sec

35. Which of the following terms refers to the posterior aspect of the body?

    a. Ventral.
    b. Ipsilateral.
    c. Lateral.
    d. Dorsal.

36. Using the Fox & Haskell model to estimate the maximum heart rate (MHR) and the percentage method to estimate the target heart rate (THR), if the patient is age 60 and engages in moderate-intensity exercise (70%), what is the patient's THR?

    a. 98
    b. 102
    c. 108
    d. 112

37. In a morbidly obese patient with excess abdominal fat, the heart may be shifted:

    a. Inferiorly and to the left
    b. Superiorly and to the right
    c. Inferiorly and to the right
    d. Superiorly and to the left

38. Which type of premature ventricular contractions (PVCs) are evident on the following EKG tracing?

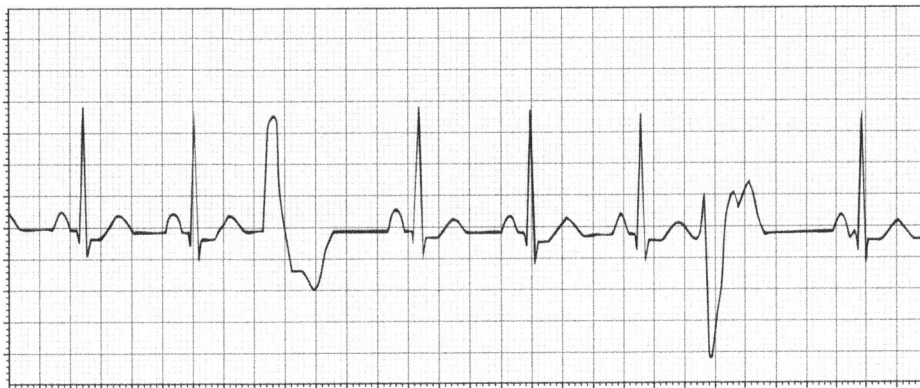

    a. Unifocal
    b. Bigeminy
    c. Couplet
    d. Multifocal

39. The EKG technician is performing an EKG exam on a patient with suspected pacemaker malfunction. What does the following EKG tracing suggest?

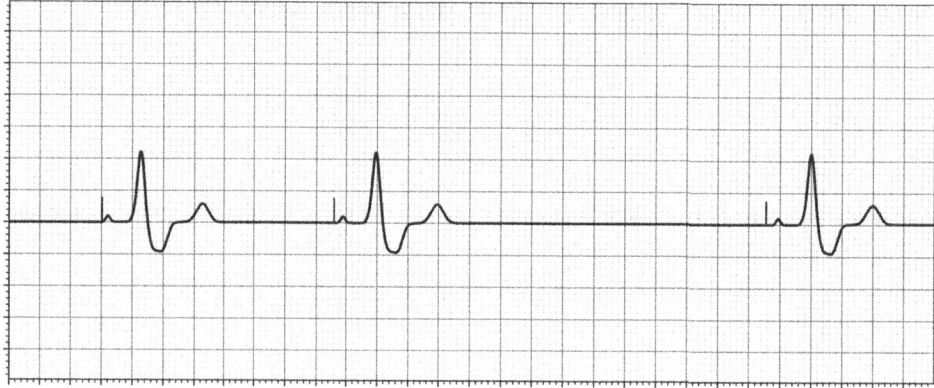

    a. Failure to sense
    b. Normal functioning
    c. Failure to capture
    d. Failure to pace

40. In the following EKG tracing, the red arrow is pointing at:

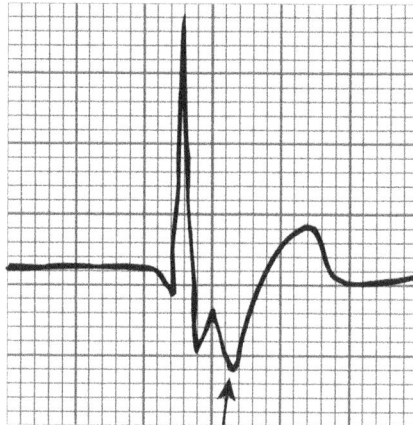

    a. ST depression
    b. Inverted P wave
    c. Inverted T wave
    d. Biphasic T wave

41. What is a normal heart rate for a 6-year-old child?

    a. 90–160
    b. 80–150
    c. 65–120
    d. 60–100

42. The rhythm in this EKG strip is best described as:

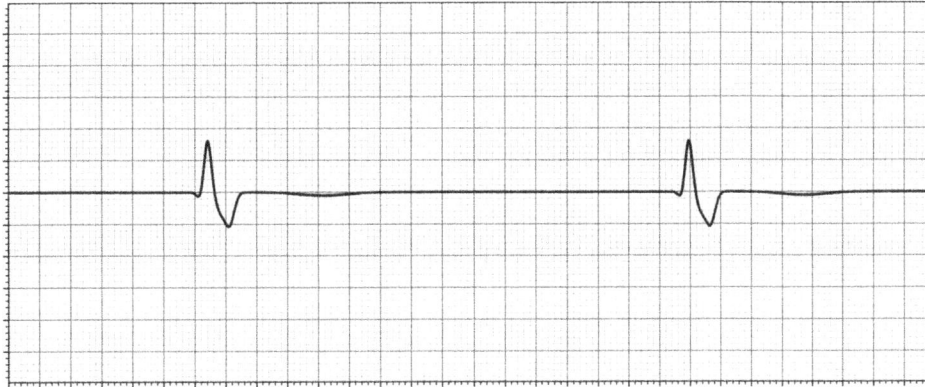

a. Agonal rhythm
b. Pulseless electrical activity
c. Sinus bradycardia
d. Third-degree heart block

43. The EKG technician must perform an EKG exam on a child hospitalized with measles. What type of precautions are required?

a. Standard alone
b. Standard and contact
c. Standard and droplet
d. Standard and airborne

44. The nipple line is used as a reference for electrode placement for children less than:

a. 6 months of age
b. 12 months of age
c. 60 lb (27 kg)
d. 90 lb (41 kg)

45. For a broken recording artifact, the first step to resolve the issue should be to:

a. Check the lead wires/cables.
b. Change the electrodes.
c. Ask the patient to stop moving.
d. Check the electrical equipment in the area.

46. If a skin prep for long-term event monitoring is needed to remove surface oils, dirt, and dead skin cells, which one of the following choices is generally the best option?

a. Mild abrasive pads (e.g., 3M Red Dot Trace Prep)
b. Dry gauze
c. Alcohol (70% isopropyl) wipes
d. Medical sandpaper or abrasive tape

47. An *artifact* is best described as a(n):

a. Error in the measurement of electrical activity
b. Normal variance in a recorded signal
c. Visual representation of a cardiac arrhythmia
d. Distortion or interference in a recorded signal

48. Which of the following is NOT a violation of the Health Insurance Portability and Accountability Act (HIPAA)?

    a. Releasing patient information to a third party without a patient signature.
    b. Talking about a patient's condition during shift change at the nursing desk to the patient's oncoming EKG technician.
    c. Throwing a medical chart in a trash can.
    d. Discussing a patient's case over social media.

49. Which type of SA block is characterized by a regular rhythm with a sudden dropped P wave?

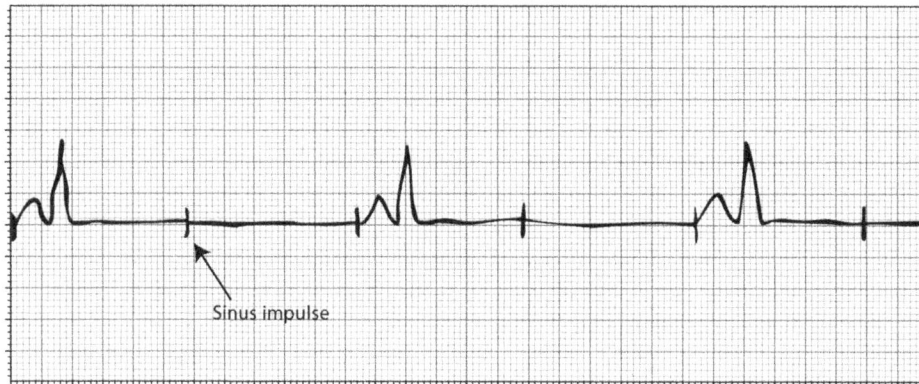

Sinus impulse

    a. First-degree SA block
    b. Second-degree SA block, type I
    c. Second-degree SA block, type II
    d. Third-degree SA block

50. If a patient is scheduled for a stress echocardiogram, what type of baseline EKG should the EKG technician anticipate will be needed?

    a. 3-lead
    b. 5-lead
    c. 7-lead
    d. 12-lead

51. If electrical conduction in the heart is blocked below the bundle of His (severe third-degree blockage), what part of the conduction system can serve as the pacemaker?

    a. SA node
    b. Purkinje fibers
    c. Bachmann's bundle
    d. AV node

52. The double-layered sac that encases the heart is the:

    a. Endocardium
    b. Myocardium
    c. Epicardium
    d. Pericardium

53. If the EKG technician has placed electrodes for an EKG on a patient with a seizure disorder and the patient experiences a seizure before the recording begins, the EKG technician should:

    a. Continue recording and note the seizure on the EKG strip.
    b. Discontinue the EKG altogether.
    c. Delay the recording until the seizure subsides.
    d. Take a recording during the seizure and another after it subsides.

54. When placing EKG strips on mounting paper for the physician to assess arrhythmias, how long should the rhythm strips typically be?

    a. 4 seconds
    b. 5 seconds
    c. 6 seconds
    d. 8 seconds

55. If a female patient who requires an EKG has very large, pendulous breasts and is unable to lift the breast tissue out of the way by herself, the EKG technician should lift the breast tissue with (the):

    a. Both hands
    b. Back of the hand
    c. Fingers
    d. Palm of the hand

56. If the EKG technician believes that the patient's heart rate is too rapid for the 25 mm/sec EKG setting, the EKG technician may change it to 50 mm/sec:

    a. If allowed by facility protocol
    b. Without further consultation
    c. Only with a physician's order
    d. Only for pediatric patients

57. In which of the following physical examination methods is a stethoscope used to listen for lung and heart sounds?

    a. Palpation
    b. Percussion
    c. Auscultation
    d. Mensuration

EKG Tech Practice Test #1

58. What is the approximate duration of the QRS complex on the EKG tracing above?

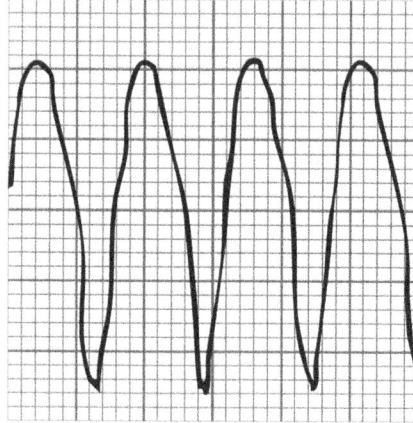

    a. 0.28 sec
    b. 0.32 sec
    c. 0.36 sec
    d. 0.40 sec

59. Following an exercise stress test, within at least how many minutes should the EKG technician expect that the patient's heart rate, respiration rate, BP, and oxygen saturation will return to baseline?

    a. 5
    b. 10
    c. 15
    d. 20

60. A patient with rapid respiratory rate has which condition?

    a. Tachycardia.
    b. Bradycardia.
    c. Tachypnea.
    d. Hypotension.

61. The EKG technician is performing an EKG exam and notes the following tracing. What is the most likely cause?

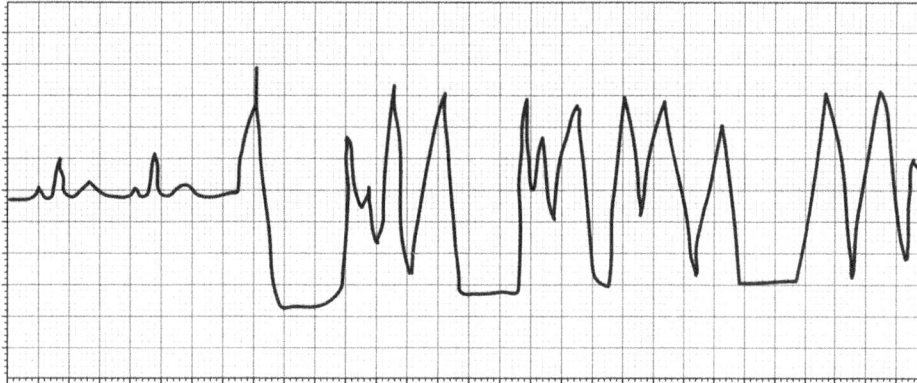

a. Broken recording
b. Muscle movement artifact
c. Ventricular fibrillation
d. Heart block

62. What type of electrolyte imbalance does a peaked T wave often indicate?

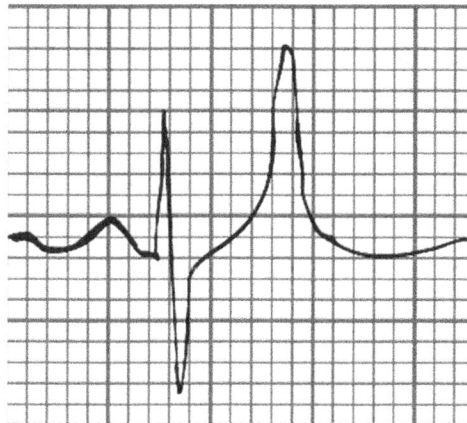

a. Hyperkalemia
b. Hypokalemia
c. Hypercalcemia
d. Hypocalcemia

63. If a patient has an above-the-knee amputation of the right leg with a 4-inch stump, the most appropriate placement for the EKG electrodes is:

a. Left lower leg and right stump
b. Left and right torso below ribs
c. Left upper leg and stump
d. Left upper leg and right torso below ribs

64. Which of the following is a violation of Health Insurance Portability and Accountability Act (HIPAA)?

   a. Discussing the patient's prognosis with his or her power of attorney.
   b. Sending a patient's records to his or her designated primary care doctor.
   c. Keeping yourself logged into the hospital computer to allow quicker documentation.
   d. Disposing of sensitive documents in a shredder.

65. What does the following EKG strip represent?

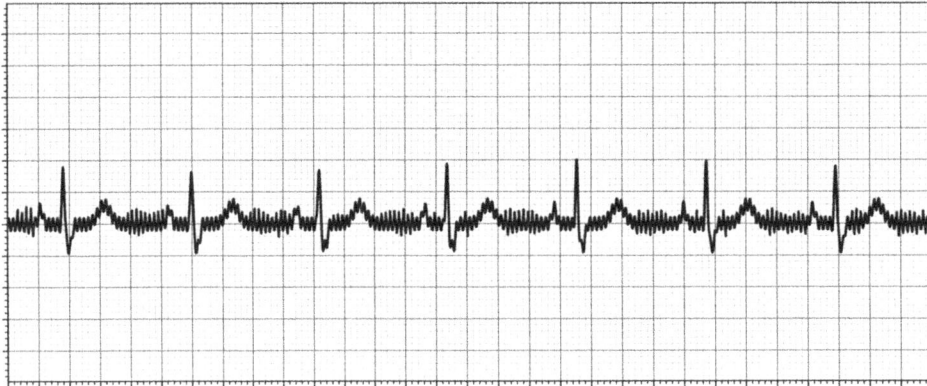

   a. Atrial flutter
   b. Atrial fibrillation
   c. Alternating current/60-cycle artifacts
   d. Poorly connected leads

66. When monitoring a patient's oxygen saturation during an exercise stress test, at what oxygen saturation level should the test be immediately stopped?

   a. ≤93%
   b. ≤90%
   c. ≤88%
   d. ≤85%

67. The EKG technician performs an EKG exam, and most of the EKG shows a normal sinus rhythm, but near the end of the EKG exam, the technician notes new abnormalities. The EKG technician should:

   a. Take a second EKG and give both to the healthcare provider.
   b. Take a second EKG and give only the second one to the healthcare provider.
   c. Mount the EKG and give it to healthcare provider.
   d. Ask the healthcare provider about whether to perform a second EKG.

68. What does the following EKG strip represent?

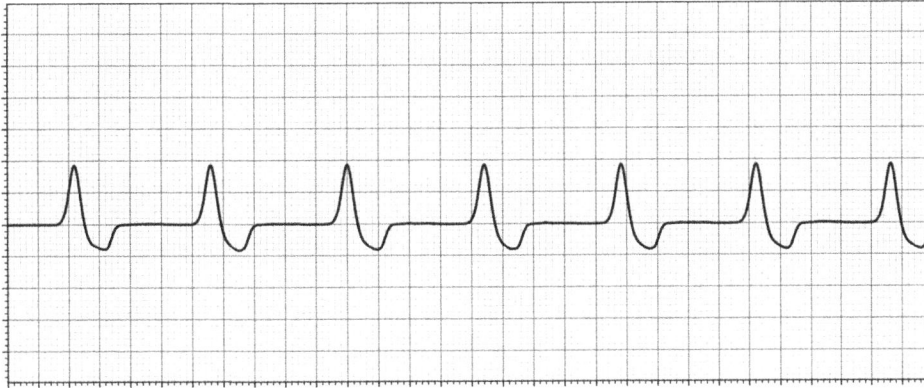

a. Ventricular escape
b. VT
c. Accelerated idioventricular rhythm
d. Junctional tachycardia with bundle branch block

69. While preparing to capture an EKG on a patient, you witness a patient suddenly collapse. You run to the patient and realize she is unconscious, does not have a pulse, and is not breathing. While someone else calls a code, you and a patient care technician begin cardiopulmonary resuscitation (CPR). At what point should you use an automated external defibrillator (AED)?

a. After one round or two minutes of CPR have been performed
b. As soon as emergency medical help arrives
c. If the patient still has no pulse after five minutes of CPR
d. As soon as possible

70. Which of the following are included in the scope of practice for EKG technicians? (Select the three [3] correct answers.)

a. Prepare patients for ambulatory monitoring.
b. Calibrate EKG equipment.
c. Recommend modification of the patient care plan.
d. Initiate basic life support.
e. Diagnose/interpret EKG results.

71. Which chamber of the heart is most responsible for the cardiac output?

a. Right atrium
b. Left atrium
c. Right ventricle
d. Left ventricle

72. Which type of lead clip is the most reliable?

a. Banana plug
b. Alligator
c. Pinch
d. Snap

73. **For posterior monitoring, electrode V8 is placed at:**
    a. Fifth intercostal space, posterior axillary line
    b. Fifth intercostal space, posterior left paraspinal line
    c. Fifth intercostal space, posterior midscapular line
    d. Fifth intercostal space, posterior paraspinal/paravertebral line

74. **A patient with an automatic implantable cardioverter-defibrillator (AICD) should generally be advised to avoid:**
    a. Microwave ovens
    b. Magnetic resonance imaging (MRI) scans
    c. Metal detectors
    d. Antitheft devices

75. **What type of tachycardia does the following EKG tracing represent?**

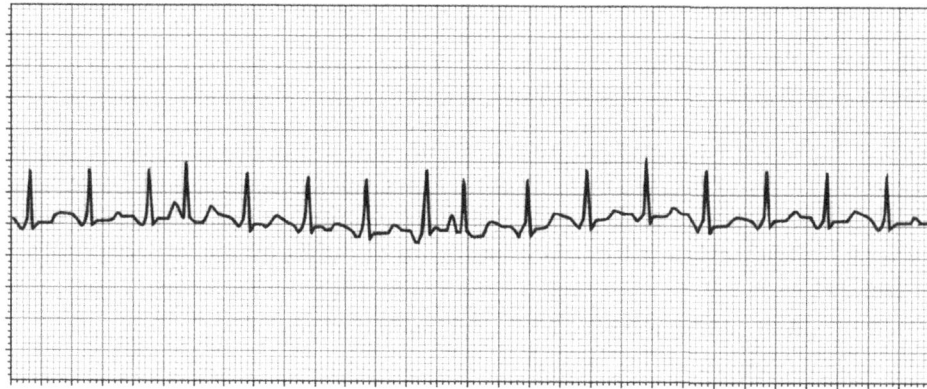

    a. Multifocal/Multiform atrial tachycardia
    b. Junctional tachycardia
    c. Sinus tachycardia
    d. Torsades de pointes

76. **If an EKG tracing shows that lead I is normal but lead III is missing, the EKG technician should suspect that the problem is with the:**
    a. LL electrode
    b. LA electrode
    c. RL electrode
    d. RA electrode

77. **When beginning an exercise test on a treadmill, the initial speed using the Bruce protocol is set at:**
    a. 1.2 mph
    b. 1.7 mph
    c. 2.5 mph
    d. 3.4 mph

78. If a patient undergoing an EKG has a cardiac arrest and the EKG technician has called for help, the EKG technician should begin cardiopulmonary resuscitation (CPR) with:

    a. Cycles of 30 compressions to 2 breaths
    b. Compressions only at a rate of 100 bpm
    c. Cycles of 15 compressions to 4 breaths
    d. Cycles of 60 compressions to 4 breaths

79. The midclavicular line usually lies:

    a. Lateral to the nipple in men
    b. Lateral to the nipple in men and women
    c. Medial to the nipple in men
    d. Medial to the nipple in men and women

80. What is the meaning of an *ectopic beat*?

    a. Contraction from an impulse not originating from the SA node
    b. Contraction originating from an impulse from the AV node
    c. Contraction originating from an impulse in the ventricles
    d. Contraction from an impulse not conducted through the ventricles

81. Which formula for determining the MHR is generally most accurate for older adults?

    a. Fox & Haskell
    b. Nes
    c. Gulati
    d. Tanaka

82. Which artery is normally palpated in the wrist to take a pulse?

    a. Popliteal.
    b. Brachial.
    c. Radial.
    d. Jugular.

83. On an EKG tracing, the J point is located:

    a. At the end of the P wave before the QRS segment
    b. Where the QRS complex transitions into the ST segment
    c. Where the T wave transitions to the P wave
    d. At the peak of the T wave

84. An exercise stress test should be immediately stopped if the patient's systolic blood pressure (BP) is greater than what minimal threshold?

    a. 180 mmHg
    b. 200 mmHg
    c. 220 mmHg
    d. 250 mmHg

85. What is the proper way to position a blood pressure cuff?

    a. Wrap the cuff loosely around the upper part of the forearm, about an inch below the elbow.
    b. Wrap the cuff snugly around the upper arm, as close to the shoulder as possible.
    c. Wrap the cuff around the elbow, just tight enough to keep it in place.
    d. Wrap the cuff snugly around the upper arm, about half an inch above the elbow.

86. Who can do cardiopulmonary resuscitation (CPR)?
   a. Physicians.
   b. Nurses.
   c. Medical Assistants.
   d. Anyone who has passed a certification course.

87. For an EKG, a woman should be asked to remove an underwire bra primarily because:
   a. It makes electrode application difficult.
   b. It may increase her discomfort during the procedure.
   c. The wire may cause artifacts.
   d. She may get an electric shock.

88. The purpose of the RL electrode in a standard 12-lead EKG is to:
   a. Generate lead IV
   b. Contribute to augmented leads
   c. Serve as a ground
   d. Generate lead VI

89. If the EKG technician is performing an EKG exam on a patient who was alert and responsive with clear speech during preparation but whose speech suddenly becomes slurred, the EKG technician should:
   a. Call for help immediately.
   b. Ask questions to further assess the patient's speech.
   c. Finish the EKG and then report the speech change to a nurse or physician.
   d. Advise the patient to take deep breaths and relax.

90. What does an Osborn, or J, wave typically indicate on an EKG tracing?
   a. Hyperkalemia
   b. Hypokalemia
   c. Hypothermia
   d. Hyperthermia

91. A transgender female patient has had breast implants. For an EKG, the electrodes should be placed:
   a. Above the implants on the upper chest
   b. On the implants
   c. Under the implants
   d. Over or under the implants as needed for correct electrode positioning

92. Before a stress test is conducted, which of the following must be readily available? (Select the three [3] correct answers.)
   a. Oxygen
   b. Blood glucose monitor
   c. External defibrillator/manual defibrillator
   d. Crash cart
   e. Continuous positive airway pressure device

93. Which of the following is NOT an acceptable method of hand-washing as part of infection control?

    a. Medical asepsis hand wash using an antimicrobial soap
    b. Medical asepsis hand wash using a non-antimicrobial soap
    c. Antibacterial wipes
    d. Alcohol-based hand rub

94. If the physician has requested a 12-lead EKG using the Lund lead system modification, this means that the limb leads are placed on the:

    a. Upper and lower torso
    b. Distal area of the limbs
    c. Proximal area of the limbs
    d. Proximal area of arms and distal area of legs

95. If an overweight male patient has very large breasts, the chest electrodes should be placed:

    a. On or under the breast, whichever is closest to the correct position
    b. On top of the breast only
    c. Under the breast only
    d. On and under the breast (make two recordings)

96. What rhythm is evident on this EKG strip?

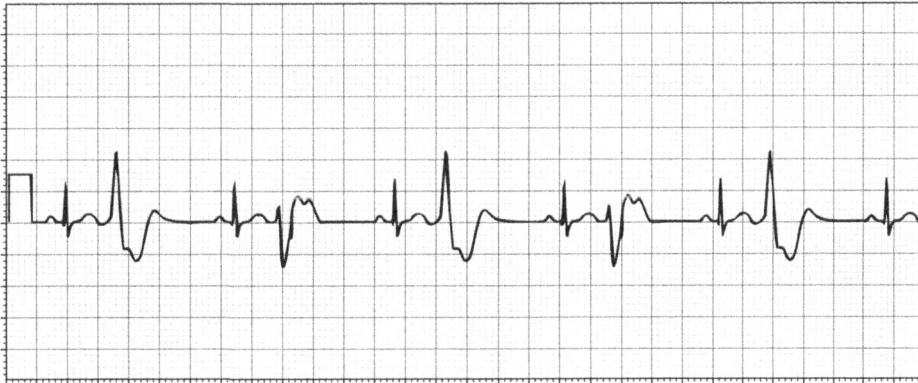

    a. AV block (Mobitz I)
    b. Atrial bigeminy
    c. Ventricular escape beats
    d. PVC and ventricular bigeminy

97. A woman in her third trimester of pregnancy is scheduled for an EKG. Her prepregnancy baseline heart rate was 82. What heart rate should the EKG technician recognize as being within the normal range for this patient during her third trimester?

    a. 62 bpm
    b. 74 bpm
    c. 86 bpm
    d. 100 bpm

98. Which of the following reflects a PR interval seen with first degree heart block?

    a. 0.12.
    b. 0.16.
    c. 0.20.
    d. 0.24.

99. What type of pacemaker malfunction does the following EKG tracing demonstrate?

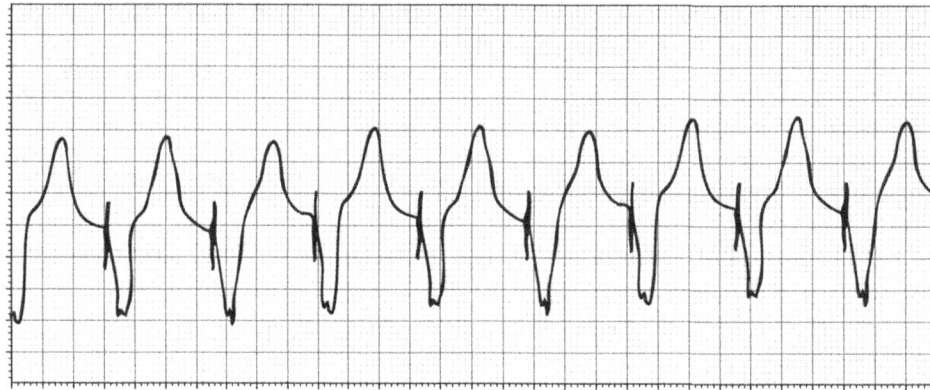

    a. Pacemaker-mediated tachycardia
    b. Runaway pacemaker
    c. Failure to sense
    d. Failure to capture

100. What is the underlying rhythm of this EKG tracing with premature atrial contractions (PACs)?

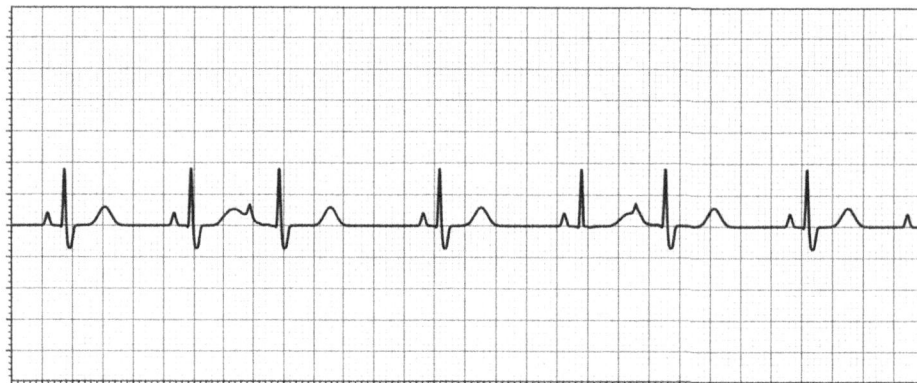

    a. Sinus rhythm
    b. Sinus bradycardia
    c. Sinus tachycardia
    d. Wandering atrial pacemaker

Answer Key and Explanations for Test #1

1. C: The Brugada sign is characterized by a coved, elevated ST segment of greater than 2 mm and a negative T wave in more than one lead of V1, V2, and V3. If coupled with specific clinical signs, such as a history of atrial fibrillation or polymorphic VT and a family history of sudden cardiac death before age 45, these signs are diagnostic for Brugada syndrome. Brugada syndrome is an inherited cardiac disorder that causes an increased risk of ventricular fibrillation and sudden cardiac death, especially in males of Asian heritage in their 30s and 40s.

2. B: Two forms of identification should always be used to verify a patient's identification. The most common method of assessing identification is through asking "What is your name and birthdate?" If the patient is wearing a wristband, this can also be checked, but the wristband should not be relied on alone. If a patient is not able to respond verbally or is confused, the information on the wristband should be verified in the patient's medical record. If the wristband contains a barcode, it should be scanned to ensure that it matches the barcode of the medical record.

3. B: First-degree heart block occurs when the electrical impulse generated by the SA node remains uninterrupted but is delayed through the AV node. First-degree heart block is usually benign. Characteristics of first-degree heart block include a P wave present for every QRS complex, a P-R interval of greater than 0.20 sec, and no missing beats. If the P-R interval extends to more than 0.30 sec, then the P wave may be hidden in the previous T wave and patients may begin to experience symptoms.

4. B: Paroxysmal SVT is sudden episodes of tachycardia originating above the ventricles because of abnormal electrical conduction in the atria or AV node. It is a dysrhythmia characterized by a regular heart rate of 150–250 bpm with abnormally shaped P waves (that may be hidden in the preceding T waves) but with a normal PR interval and a normal QRS complex. The electrical discharge can originate anywhere above the bifurcation of the bundle of His. Onset is usually abrupt, and termination may be followed by a brief period of asystole. Some degree of AV block is also commonly observed.

5. D: When interpreting an EKG tracing, if waves or complexes represent the same electrical event but are different in appearance, this variation is referred to as polymorphic or multifocal. *Poly-* means many and *-morphic* means shape. Polymorphic is the opposite of monomorphic, in which each wave or complex has the same shape and appearance. Polymorphic appearances may result from electrolyte imbalances, ischemia, ventricular fibrillation, torsades de pointes, or QT prolongation. A polymorphic wave or complex is more unstable than a monomorphic one.

6. C: Both the looping memory event recorder and the postevent recorder require the patient to activate the device by pushing a button, so these devices are not useful for a patient who has silent arrhythmias or is generally unaware of symptoms. The autotriggered event recorder uses built-in algorithms to continuously monitor the heart and automatically detect and record abnormal heart rhythms, such as atrial fibrillation, tachycardia, bradycardia, pauses, and ventricular tachycardia (VT). The device stores EKG data from before, during, and after the event.

7. A, C, E: Angina is pain caused by narrowing of the coronary arteries resulting in cardiac ischemia. Angina may be experienced differently. The classic indications of angina are pain and pressure or tightness in the chest that radiates to the left shoulder and left arm, but some patients complain of pain in other areas, such as in the right shoulder and arm, the neck, and the lower jaw (common in women). Additionally, some patients may experience back pain between the shoulder blades (common in women, the elderly, and individuals with diabetes).

8. A: Atrial flutter is characterized by a rapid heart rate and repeated flutter waves instead of distinct P waves. Atrial flutter is a type of SVT resulting from a reentrant circuit within the atria that leads to atrial rates of 250–350 bpm with a ventricular rate of approximately 150 bpm. The electrical conduction is organized and predictable. Patients may experience atrial flutter as palpitations and may experience shortness of breath and dizziness. Those with coronary artery disease may have chest discomfort or angina.

9. A: Leads aVR, aVL, and aVF are the augmented leads that use the same three electrodes as leads I, II, and III, but they are unipolar leads, using a single electrode as the positive pole:

- aVR (augmented vector right): RA electrode, focuses on the right atrium and base of the right ventricle
- aVL (augmented vector left): LA electrode, focuses on the high lateral wall of the left ventricle
- aVF (augmented vector foot): LL electrode, focuses on the inferior heart wall

The leads are labeled as "augmented" because the EKG machine enhances the signal.

10. A: An open-ended question requires an answer with some detailed explanation or depth. A closed or a direct question only requires one-word answers such as yes or no.

11. B: This EKG tracing is typical of left bundle branch block. The QRS duration is ≥120 ms. The QRS complex widens because activation of the left ventricle is delayed.

- Lead V1: The QRS complex is negative with a W appearance and a dominant S wave. The R wave may be small, or there may be no preceding R wave.
- Lead V6: The QRS complex is broad and positive. The R wave is broad with a notched M appearance.

12. B: For a nuclear stress test, a baseline 12-lead EKG is obtained, and then continuous monitoring is done during the exercise portion of the test. After the exercise is completed, repeat 12-lead EKG exams are performed at 5, 10, and 15 minutes to assess the heart's recovery and to detect any persistent cardiac abnormalities. For example, ST depression may occur during exercise if the blood flow to some areas of the heart is inadequate. If this persists, it can indicate severe coronary artery disease. Some arrhythmias, such as VT and atrial fibrillation, may be more evident during the recovery phase.

13. C: This EKG strip shows an accelerated idioventricular rhythm (AIVR) with a heart rate of 56 bpm. The QRS complex represents ventricular contraction. The QRS complex is generally measured from the first downward deflection of the Q wave, but this downward deflection may be absent, as in this example. The QRS complex is prolonged at 0.18 sec (the normal QRS duration is 0.06–0.10 sec), and the P wave is absent. If the complex is wide, this is an indication of abnormal conduction.

14. A: The normal duration and amplitude of different components of the EKG waveform:

Component	Duration	Amplitude
P wave	<0.12 s	≤2.5 mm (lead II)
P-R interval	0.12–0.20 s	—
PR segment	0.08–0.12 s	—
QRS complex	0.06–0.10 se	Limb leads ≤5 mm, precordial leads ≤10 mm
Q-T interval	Men ≤0.44 s, Women ≤0.46 s	—
ST segment	Isoelectric, not usually measured in seconds	—
T wave	Varies with heart rate	Limb leads ≤5 mm, precordial leads ≤10 mm

15. D: Sending a patient's medical records to their primary care doctor's office is not a HIPAA violation. It is necessary to maintain a continuity of care after a patient has seen a specialist for a new problem or has been recently been hospitalized.

16. A: The chief complaint section should be a few words that summarize why the patient is in the hospital or clinic. Habits such as drug or alcohol use or type of employment belong in the social history. Precipitating or alleviating factors belong in the history of present illness section.

17. B: If the exercise stress test is causing joint pain when the incline increases, then the incline may need to be modified, such as by use of the modified Bruce protocol. If the pain is severe or if the patient is unable to tolerate even a modified protocol, then the test should be stopped. The EKG technician should note and document at which point the patient complained of pain and the circumstances and note any changes in vital signs. If a patient is unable to tolerate the exercise stress test, he or she may need to have a pharmacological stress test.

18. A: A pulse rate of 70 beats per minute is considered a normal pulse rate for an adult (range 60-80 beats per minute). However, in infants and children this would be considered too low, because average normal pulse rates steadily decline from birth through infancy and childhood. The other choices are abnormalities. Bradycardia is a pulse rate of less than 60 beats per minute. Tachycardia is a pulse rate of more than 100 beats per minute. Arrhythmia is any abnormal electrical activity in the heart, resulting in alteration of the interval between pulsations.

19. B: The brachial artery can be palpated on the ventral surface of the arm anterior to the elbow. The blood pressure cuff or sphygmomanometer and a stethoscope can be used to help measure blood pressure by auscultating Korotkoff sounds. Systolic pressure is registered as the pressure at which the sounds are first heard, and diastolic as the pressure at which they disappear.

20. D: Vasovagal syncope is triggered by the parasympathetic nervous system in response to a trigger, such as anxiety, overheating, or prolonged standing. Vasodilation causes hypotension and the heart rate to slow (reducing cardiac output). This results in insufficient blood to the brain and dizziness. Because the patient is at risk of falling, the EKG technician should immediately assist him to sit and, if able, to lie down. If these symptoms result from vasovagal syncope, then the patient should feel better within seconds to a few minutes. The EKG technician should notify the supervisor and assess the patient's vital signs.

21. C: If a patient speaks little or no English, chances are he or she will not be able to read it either. Speaking slowly so that the translator receives all of the information being given, using hand gestures, or drawing pictures may help facilitate communication.

22. D: The delta wave appears as a slurring of the upstroke of the QRS syndrome, which results in a shortened P-R interval (<0.12 sec) and a widened QRS complex (>0.10 sec). This finding is characteristic of Wolff-Parkinson-White syndrome—a congenital cardiac disorder that affects the electrical conduction in the heart. An extra or accessory pathway connects the atria and ventricles, bypassing the AV node. This cause preexcitation of the ventricles and an increased risk of tachyarrhythmias.

23. D: A living will is a written document that specifies what a patient would like to be done if he becomes unable to make healthcare decisions for himself. In a living will, the patient can express his wishes about what life-prolonging treatments he wants or does not want under various circumstances. It is a document focused on healthcare decisions, not on the patient's material assets.

24. A: First-degree AV block is a conduction delay between the atria and the AV node or His-Purkinje system in the ventricles. The rhythm is regular with no dropped beats, and a P wave is present before each QRS complex; however, the P-R interval is prolonged to greater than 0.20 sec (five small boxes). The QRS complexes are normal and remain narrow (<0.12 sec). First-degree AV block is usually benign if it is asymptomatic. Pacing is not generally required unless the P-R interval exceeds 0.30 sec.

25. B: Lead II aligns best with the natural depolarization of the heart, so it is used most often for continuous cardiac monitoring and rhythm analysis. Lead II produces well-defined, upright P waves; well-defined QRS complexes; and clear T waves because it follows the depolarization of the heart from the SA node, through the atria, to the AV node, and down the bundle of His and Purkinje fibers. Lead II shows atrial activity, conduction abnormalities, and ventricular rhythms.

26. B: The skin consists of three layers: the epidermis (outer layer), made up of squamous epithelium, keratin, and melanin; the dermis (middle layer), which contains the blood vessels, nerve endings, glands, and some connective tissue; and the hypodermis (deepest layer), with subcutaneous connective and adipose tissue. Integumentary is the inclusive name for the system of the skin and its connected structures, like hair, nails, nerve endings, and oil and sweat glands.

27. C: Children are typically frightened of any medical procedure, especially if they fear that the procedure will hurt, so it is especially important to reassure children that the EKG exam does not hurt and takes only a few minutes. The EKG technician should explain the EKG in simple terms and should avoid any type of medical jargon, such as "electrodes" or "leads" but should instead use terms the child may be familiar with, such as "stickers" and "cords." The EKG should encourage the child to ask questions about the EKG before beginning the procedure.

28. A: If a patient grimaces during an exercise stress test, the EKG technician should ask if the patient is having discomfort to determine if the grimace is because of exertion, musculoskeletal pain, chest pain, or another issue. The EKG technician should also check the vital signs and oxygen saturation for changes that may indicate cardiac ischemia. If the patient reports that the grimacing is due to exertion, then it is generally safe to continue the test and monitor the patient carefully.

29. A: Digoxin is a medication used to treat heart failure, atrial flutter, and atrial fibrillation. It slows the heart rate and the rate of conduction through the AV node. Patients who are receiving digoxin therapy may have the following EKG changes:

- Sloping ST depression (i.e., the appearance of a reverse checkmark)
- T wave changed: flattened, inverted, or biphasic, peaking of the terminal part of the T wave
- Prominent U waves
- J point depression
- P-R interval may be prolonged (up to 0.24 sec)

30. B: Atrial fibrillation occurs with the generation of multiple simultaneous electrical impulses in the atria, resulting in rapid and chaotic depolarizations. Characteristics include an irregular rhythm with irregular R-R intervals with no predictable pattern, an absence of distinct P waves (replaced by fibrillatory [f] waves[in leads II, III, aVF, and V1]), an atrial rate of 350–600 bpm (but not all impulses are conducted through the AV node), and a ventricular rate of 80–100 bpm.

31. C: Hypocalcemia is characterized by a prolonged ST segment and a prolonged QT interval, while hypercalcemia is characterized by a shortened ST segment and a widened T wave. Because calcium is needed for contraction of the heart muscle, hypocalcemia weakens the contractions and can lead to bradycardia and hypotension. Hypercalcemia is characterized by a shortened Q-T interval and a shortened ST segment. Hypercalcemia initially leads to increased contractility, but high levels can impair the ability of the heart muscle to relax and may lead to hypertension, ventricular and atrial arrhythmias, AV block, and asystole.

32. A: With a wandering baseline, the baseline moves gradually up and down over multiple leads. This can result in misalignment of the waveforms. A wandering baseline is often caused by patient movement or deep breathing, so the first step is to ask the patient to lie still and to breathe normally. If the problem persists, the technician should check the electrodes' placement to ensure that they are not over bony or uneven surfaces and are not loose, and that the conducting gel has not dried out. In some cases, lead wires may be pulling on the electrodes or may be faulty.

33. C: If a neonate is crying and moving about, it is impossible to get an accurate EKG. The EKG technician should ask if there are comfort measures, such as a sucralose pacifier, available to help soothe the infant. The EKG technician should make sure that the infant is in a cot with overhead heating, if possible, to reduce heat loss and discomfort. Swaddling may also comfort the child. If necessary, the electrodes can be placed and then recordings made when the child calms.

34. A: The P-R interval is the duration between atrial polarization (i.e., the beginning of the P wave) and ventricular depolarization (i.e., the beginning of the QRS complex or from the beginning of the R wave if no Q wave deflection is present). In this tracing, there are approximately six small boxes comprising the P-R interval, which is a duration of approximately 0.24 sec (6 × 0.04). The normal range for the P-R interval is 0.12–0.20 sec, so the P-R interval is prolonged. This is an indication of heart block.

35. D: The dorsum of an object refers to the posterior or back part. Ventral or anterior means the front of something. Ipsilateral means the same side. Lateral is next to or on the side of something.

36. D: The maximum heart rate (MHR) is the upper limit for the heart rate the patient can achieve during maximum exertion, while the target heart rate (THR) is the ideal rate for the patient based on the intensity of exercise. This patient is age 60, and the patient's exercise intensity level is 70%. The calculation is as follows:

Fox & Haskell: 220 – age = MHR

- 220 – 60 = 160 MHR

Percentage method for THR: MHR × exercise intensity level

- 160 × 0.70 = 112 THR

The patient's THR is 112.

37. D: If a patient is morbidly obese with excess abdominal fat, the visceral fat may apply pressure to the heart and over time shift the heart superiorly and to the left. Because of this, the electrodes may need to be positioned higher. For example, V1 and V2 may need to be at the second or third intercostal space rather than the fourth and V3 through V6 may need to may need to be moved laterally. In some cases, all precordial leads are placed one to two intercostal spaces higher to compensate for the increased elevation of the diaphragm.

38. D: This EKG tracing is an example of multifocal premature ventricular contractions (PVCs) because the PVCs vary in appearance with different QRS shapes (unlike unifocal PVCs). Other characteristics include no P wave or P-R interval associated with the PVC, and an irregular rhythm when the PVC occurs. With bigeminy, a PVC occurs after every normal heartbeat. Couplets are when two PVCs occur, one after another. In healthy individuals, isolated multiform PVCs are usually benign, but in the present of heart disease, they may indicate an increased risk of sudden cardiac death or ventricular tachyarrhythmias.

39. D: With failure to pace, the pacemaker spikes on the EKG tracing are absent when the heart rate is slow and there is no evidence of pacemaker activity. The tracing will only show the underlying rhythm and may indicate bradycardia or even asystole in severe cases. Causes of failure to pace include depletion of the battery, a broken or displaced lead preventing delivery of the impulse, internal circuit failure, electromagnetic interference (e.g., MRI, electrocautery, defibrillators), or incorrect programming (e.g., sensitivity settings).

40. B: With retrograde depolarization, instead of an electrical impulse generating from the SA node in an up-and-down and right-to-left direction, the impulse originates from below the atria and travels in reverse to depolarize the atria. This results in an inverted P wave in leads in which the deflection is usually positive. Depending on where the impulse originates, the inverted P wave may appear before the QRS complex; it may be hidden within the QRS complex; or it may appear, as in this illustration, after the QRS complex.

41. C: Normal vital signs are dependent on age, as follows:

Age	Heart Rate	Blood Pressure	Respirations
Newborn	100–180	No standardized measure	30–60
≤12 months	90–160	60–90/30–60	30–60
1–3 years	80–150	80–110/50–80	22–40
3–5 years	70–140	80–110/50–80	22–40
6–12 years	65–120	90–120/60–80	18–30
13–18 years	60–100	100–130/60–85	12–20
18+ years	60–100	90–120/60–80	12–20
60+ years	60–100	110–140/60–90	12–20

42. A: Agonal rhythm is often the last rhythm seen before cardiac arrest as the heart struggles. It is a cardiac emergency and is characterized by an extremely slow heart rate (< 20 bpm), absent P waves, and a wide QRS complex with bizarre morphology. Agonal rhythm is not a shockable rhythm and typically leads to pulseless electrical activity, so immediate intervention is essential. The agonal rhythm is typically an indication of severe cardiac hypoxia. Causes of agonal rhythm include severe hypoxia, massive trauma or loss of blood, severe electrolyte imbalance, and drug overdose (e.g., fentanyl and other opioids).

43. D: Standard precautions are used with all patients; however, additional precautions may be necessary. Measles is an airborne disease; therefore, airborne precautions are required. The patient should be in a negative-pressure room with the air being filtered. The door to the room must remain closed. To enter the room, the EKG technician should wear an N95 or higher level respirator that has been fit-tested as well as a gown and gloves. If there is a risk of fluid exposure, the EKG technician should also wear eye protection. The technician should wash the hands both before and after administering the EKG.

44. D: With infants and children less than 90 pounds or 41 kilograms, it is not always possible to accurately assess rib spaces. For these children, the nipple line is used for reference rather than rib spaces:

- V1: On the nipple line, right of the sternum
- V2: On the nipple line, left of the sternum
- V3: Midway between V2 and V4
- V4: Below the nipple line, at the midclavicular line
- V5. The same level as V4 at the anterior axillary line
- V6: The same level as V4 and V5 at the midaxillary line

45. A: If a broken recording artifact appears on the EKG tracing, the EKG technician should check the lead wires/cables because frayed or damaged lead wires is the most common cause of a broken recording. The pins at the cable end of the lead wire may be loose or damaged. A broken recording can also occur if the connections are loose or if the electrodes are dirty or are in poor contact with the skin. The EKG technician should always check all of the lead wires and connections before beginning the EKG.

46. A: Mild abrasive pads, such as 3M Red Dot Trace Prep, and pumice-containing skin gels, such as Nuprep gel, are effective at removing dirt, surface oils, and dead skin cells but are gentle enough that they generally do not cause irritation. Soap and water are also effective but may leave residual moisture. Dry gauze removes only surface dirt, while alcohol wipes remove surface oil and dirt but not dead skin cells. Stronger skin prep materials, such as medical sandpaper or abrasive tape, are very effective but may cause skin irritation.

47. D: An artifact is a distortion or interference in a recorded signal that affects the accuracy of the recording. In medicine, this definition can apply to medical imaging, electroencephalograms, and laboratory tests as well as EKGs. Typical artifacts found on EKG tracings include:

- Somatic tremor: Caused by involuntary muscle movement or voluntary muscle contractions, shivering, tremors, anxiety
- Electrical/60-cycle interference: Caused by electrical sources in the vicinity
- Wandering baseline: Caused by loose or dry electrodes, improper electrode placement, or inadequate skin preparation
- Broken recording: Caused by loose, disconnected, or damaged lead wires or cables

48. B: Talking about a case to providers involved in the patient's care at the nurses station is not a HIPAA violation. Shift change is a common time for this type of discussion. Taking about a case in public areas such as elevators or cafeterias, where individuals that are not involved in the care of the patient, would be a violation of patient privacy. Releasing medical information without consent, throwing away a chart in a non-designated trash bin, or talking about a case on social media are also violations.

49. C: Second-degree SA block, type II, is characterized by a regular rhythm with a sudden dropped P wave, resulting in a pause because no QRS complex is generated. The SA node generates an electrical impulse, but some fails to exit the SA node, resulting in P waves being intermittently missed. Second-degree SA block, type II is more concerning than second-degree SA block, type I because it can progress to third-degree SA block or asystole.

50. D: For a stress echocardiogram, generally a 12-lead EKG is done to record baseline rhythms and to detect any cardiac abnormalities. Once this is completed, then a 3- or 5-lead configuration is used during the exercise phase of the echocardiogram so that the precordial area is clear for the ultrasound probe. If a treadmill or cyclometer is used, then the images are obtained before and immediately after peak exertion. With the dobutamine stress echocardiogram, images are taken at multiple stages: baseline, early stress (low dose), peak stress (increased dose), and post stress (after infusion).

51. B: If the AV node has a first-degree blockage (Mobitz I), the SA node is able to pace the heart at a normal rate (60–100 bpm) and typically no intervention is required. If the block is early third-degree (Mobitz II), then the bundle of His takes over the pacemaker function, but the heart rate is 40–60 bpm, so a pacemaker may be required. If the block is severe third-degree and below the bundle of His, then the Purkinje fibers can take over, but the heart rate ranges from 20–40 bpm, so the patient requires a pacemaker.

52. D: The heart comprises three layers and a double-layered sac that encases it, the pericardium. Layers of the heart are as follows:

- Endocardium: Thin smooth inner lining provides a protective barrier
- Myocardium: Thick muscle tissue responsible for heart contractions
- Epicardium: Thin outer protective membrane
- Pericardium: Comprises two layers, the parietal pericardium (inner surface) and the visceral pericardium (the outer layer)

53. C: If a patient experiences a seizure during an EKG, this will result in somatic artifacts that can make it difficult to correctly interpret the heart's electrical activity, so the best solution is to delay the recording until the seizure subsides. Additionally, seizures can alter the underlying heart rate and rhythm (e.g., tachycardia, bradycardia, Q-T interval changes and ST-segment shifts), and these changes may not reflect the patient's normal baseline findings. During a seizure, the focus should be on protecting the patient from injury and protecting the airway and oxygenation.

54. C: In order to assess arrhythmias, a 6-second EKG strip is usually needed. If multiple leads are to be mounted, they should be arranged in order and placed horizontally on the mounting sheet. The EKG strips may need to be trimmed, but it is important to ensure that important waveforms are visible. The strips should be labeled with the patient's name, ID, and date, lead placement, and any important clinical details, such as "during episodes of chest pain."

55. B: Large, pendulous breasts can pose a challenge to electrode placement for an EKG, but the electrodes should be placed under, not on, the breast. The EKG technician should explain the need to move the breast tissue and ask the patient to lift the breast if possible. If the patient is unable to do so, then the EKG technician should use the back of the hand to slide under the breast and then lift and push upward.

56. A: The standard EKG exam is performed at a speed of 25 mm/s. If the patient's heart rate is very rapid, a rate of 50 mm/s may make the EKG easier to interpret. However, the EKG technician should consult with a physician before changing the speed unless facility protocol allows for the EKG technician to adjust the speed when necessary. In some cases, both an EKG at 25 mm/s may be taken as well as one at a speed of 50 mm/s so that the healthcare provider can compare them.

57. C: This examination is auscultation. Palpation is the use of touch to feel for things like body parts, masses, and skin texture. Percussion is tapping with the fingers or a percussion hammer to listen for characteristic dull or hollow sounds. Mensuration is taking measurements such as height, weight, and circumference of a body part. Other examination methods include observation of things like symmetry and posture, and manipulation to check for range of motion.

58. B: The QRS complex on the EKG tracing shown is approximately 0.32 sec (8 small boxes × 0.04 sec = 0.32 sec). This is an example of VT with a wide QRS complex because the QRS complex is greater than 0.12 sec (three small boxes). The heart rate is approximately 200 bpm, and P waves and the P-R interval are absent. Wide-complex VT may originate in the ventricles or above the ventricles with abnormal conduction. Wide-complex VT is usually regular.

59. C: Following an exercise stress test, the heart rate, respiration rate, BP, and oxygen saturation should return to baseline within 15 minutes because the parasympathetic nervous system takes over from the sympathetic nervous system. The systolic BP usually returns close to baseline within 5–10 minutes. During the first minute, the heart rate should decrease ≥12 bpm during active recovery (light slow-down exercise) or ≥18 bpm with passive recovery and ≥22 bpm in the second minute. Typically, complete recovery ranges from 5–10 minutes. The respiratory rate should slowly decrease and return to baseline within <15 minutes. The oxygen saturation usually remains stable.

60. C: Tachypnea is an elevated respiratory rate. A normal respiratory rate is 12–20 breaths per minute. Tachycardia is an elevated heart rate. Bradypnea is a decreased respiratory rate. Hypotension is low blood pressure.

61. A: This EKG tracing is an example of a broken recording. That is, there is an interruption or loss of signal for a period of time that results in the stylus going from side to side in search of the signal. A common cause is a broken or frayed lead wire, so the EKG technician should always check the wires when setting up the machine. An actual cardiac event will apear in all leads, while a broken recording will appear only in the affected leads.

62. A: A peaked T wave is often an indication of hyperkalemia, which is a life-threatening electrolyte imbalance that occurs with potassium levels greater than 5 mEq/L. The T waves are typically tall (>10 mm in precordial leads and >5 mm in limb leads) narrow, and pointed ("tented") as well as symmetrical with a sharp upslope and downslope. The peaked T waves are best observed in precordial leads V1 to V4. The Q-T interval may be shortened as well. As the potassium level increases, the P-R interval is prolonged, and the P wave flattens, progressing to a wide, bizarre QRS complex.

63. B: Because the patient's right leg stump is so short, only 4 inches, the best placement is on the patient's right and left torso, below the ribs. If the stump were longer, then the electrodes could be placed either on the torso or on the right stump and upper left leg. In whatever position is selected, the electrodes should mirror each other. Thus, it would not be appropriate to apply one electrode to a leg and the other to the torso or to apply electrodes to different positions on the legs.

64. C: Not logging off a computer properly exposes patients' sensitive information to others. Discussing the case with someone other than a patient's designated representative, sending patient records to physicians not directly involved in the patient's care, and improperly disposing of sensitive documents are other forms of HIPAA violations.

65. C: Electrical alternating current/60-cycle artifacts may show up on the EKG as a constant, repetitive, fuzzy waveform of varying amplitudes. Typically, the QRS and T waves can easily be identified despite the artifacts, although with high-frequency alternating current, they may be obscured. The spikes are usually vertical and affect all leads. Electrical interference can result from nearby power cords, electrical devices, an improperly grounded EKG machine, loose electrodes, cellphones, or fluorescent lights.

66. C: Oxygen saturation levels are monitored carefully during stress testing and should generally stay above 94%. If mild desaturation occurs (90–93%) but the patient is asymptomatic, the stress test can generally continue with careful monitoring. Clinically significant hypoxia occurs with levels <90%, and the healthcare provider may consider stopping if the patient is symptomatic, although some patients may be able to tolerate this level. An oxygen saturation level of 88% or below indicates severe hypoxia, and the test should be stopped immediately unless supplementary oxygen is provided.

67. D: Generally, unless facility protocol specifically allows the EKG technician to make decisions about second EKGs, if the technician notes abnormalities near the end of the EKG while the rest of the tracing is normal, he or she should ask the healthcare provider about performing a second EKG. While the EKG technician is not responsible for diagnosing, if he or she sees something on the EKG, such as an ST elevation, that may indicate a serious health concern, it is the responsibility of the technician to immediately notify the healthcare provider to determine if a repeat EKG is warranted.

68. C: Accelerated idioventricular rhythm (AIVR) is characterized by:

- Heart rate between 50 and 100 bpm
- Regular or only slightly irregular rhythm
- Wide QRS complex (≥120 ms)

AIVR can be mistaken for ventricular tachycardia (VT), which is typically faster than 120 bpm. VT is life-threatening, whereas AIVR is typically benign and ends without intervention. AIVR is common after reperfusion therapy and occurs in almost a third of patients. Other triggers for AIVR include potassium imbalance, drug toxicity (e.g., digoxin, flecainide, propafenone), cardiomyopathy, and after a cardiac arrest with successful resuscitation.

69. D: Because you witnessed the collapse of the patient, the automated external defibrillator (AED) should be used as soon as possible. The AED will evaluate the patient's heart rhythm while cardiopulmonary resuscitation (CPR) is being performed, so CPR can be continued while the AED pads are being applied if there is more than one responder present. The AED will give step-by-step instructions and indicate whether the patient needs to be shocked or whether CPR alone should be continued. If a patient is found unconscious and the collapse was not witnessed, two minutes or one round of CPR should be performed before using the AED.

70. A, B, D: The scope of practice for EKG technicians covers the technical and procedural aspects of cardiac monitoring, including such things as preparing patients for ambulatory monitoring, calibrating and maintaining EKG equipment, and initiating basic life support in emergent situations. However, the EKG technician cannot recommend modifications of the patient care plan or diagnose or interpret EKG results, although the technician should recognize normal and abnormal heart rhythms and alert healthcare professionals (e.g., nurse, doctor) when abnormalities occur.

71. D: The heart chamber most responsible for cardiac output is the left ventricle because it pumps the blood into the aorta and into the general systemic circulation. The cardiac output is determined by the heart rate times the stroke volume (the amount of blood that is ejected with each beat). The average volume of blood in the left ventricle when it is filled is 120–130 mL. The ejection fraction is the percentage that is expelled with each contraction, normally 50–70%. The stroke volume is the actual volume that is expelled, usually ranging from 60–100 mL.

72. D: There are four different types of lead clips: Banana plug (used in older machines), alligator, pinch, and snap. The snap lead clip is the most reliable and most widely used because it provides a stable connection that is not as likely as other clips to accidentally detach. Because the snap clip is secured to the electrode, this results in minimal motion artifacts. Additionally, most modern EKG machines use disposable electrodes, and the snap clip is compatible with most disposable electrodes. Snap clips are quick and easy to apply and remove.

73. C: Posterior EKG electrode placement is used with suspicion of posterior myocardial infarction or other need to assess the posterior heart, such as when there is ST depression or tall broad R waves in V1 through V3. Standard 12-lead electrode placement is used on the anterior chest for limb leads and V1 through V4, although V4 may be omitted. Leads V5 and V6 are typically omitted, but V6 may be included. Posterior placement includes:

- V7: Fifth intercostal space, posterior axillary line
- V8: Fifth intercostal space, posterior midscapular line
- V9: Fifth intercostal space, posterior left paraspinal/paravertebral line

74. B: A patient with an automatic implantable cardioverter-defibrillator (AICD) should generally be advised to avoid magnetic resonance imaging (MRI) scans because of the potential for harm to the patient or to the device. However, some centers have successfully done MRIs on patients with AICDs when the MRI was deemed essential, such as with suspected brain tumors. In some cases, the threshold for pacing changed or the device required reprogramming; however, no deaths or severe injuries have been associated with MRIs in patients with AICDs. Patients should avoid prolonged exposure to metal detectors and antitheft devices, but microwave ovens should cause no problems.

75. A: Multifocal/multiform atrial tachycardia is a type of SVT originating from different areas within the atria, resulting in various P wave morphologies, which are present but inconsistent in shape. The heart rate is usually greater than 100 bpm, and the P-P intervals, P-R intervals, and R-R intervals are irregular. The QRS complex tends to be narrow unless there is also a bundle branch block or other abnormality. The most common cause of this condition is pulmonary disorder (e.g., chronic obstructive pulmonary disease, pulmonary embolism, pneumonia, hypoxia, hypercapnia).

76. A: Both the LA and LL electrodes are involved in leads I and III. Since lead I is normal but lead III is missing, the EKG technician should suspect that the problem lies with the LL electrode, which is the positive electrode for lead III. Troubleshooting involves checking the electrode to determine if it is properly attached with good skin contact and the conductive gel is not dried out. If the electrode is all right, then the problem may be with a frayed or broken lead wire or an incorrect lead configuration setting on the EKG machine.

77. B: The Bruce protocol is the one most commonly used for exercise stress testing, although a modified version exists for patients with low exercise tolerance, and the Naughton protocol is used for patients after myocardial infarction and for those with severe deconditioning. The Bruce protocol for exercise test on a treadmill:

Stage	Speed (mph)	Incline (%)	Minutes
1	1.7	10%	0–3
2	2.5	12%	3–6
3	3.4	14%	6–9
4	4.2	16%	9–12
5	5.0	18%	12–15
6	5.5	20%	15–18
7	6.0	22%	18–21

78. A: An EKG technician should be trained in basic life support for healthcare professionals because many patients have underlying cardiac disease. Basic life support for healthcare professionals requires performing CPR with cycles of 30 compressions and two breaths until the automated external defibrillator (AED) or other defibrillator arrives. If the rhythm is shockable, a shock is provided and CPR is resumed immediately for 2 minutes and the rhythm is checked again. If the rhythm is nonshockable, then CPR is resumed immediately for 2 minutes and then the rhythm checked again. These cycles continue until resolution.

79. C: The midclavicular line usually lies medial to the nipple in men, but this is not a reliable guide for females because of differences in the size and shape of the breasts. Additionally, if the male is obese or has enlarged breasts, this may also not be reliable, so the EKG technician should use the clavicle as a reference point rather than the nipple. In men, the nipple is usually located at the fourth intercostal space, but it may be lower or may displaced laterally in females.

80. A: An ectopic beat is a contraction resulting from an impulse that does not originate from the SA node but from some other area of the heart, such as the AV node or the ventricles. Different types of ectopic beats include premature atrial ectopic beats, premature junctional contractions, and PVCs. Ectopic beats may present with different patterns: bigeminy, trigeminy, couplets, triplets, salvos (i.e., three or more PVCs lasting less than 30 seconds), and sustained (i.e., PVCs lasting more than 30 seconds).

81. D: The Tanaka formula (2001) for determining the maximum heart rate (MHR) was based on a meta-analysis of 18,000 older adults that showed that the heart rate usually decreases by approximately 0.7 beats per year, while the Fox & Haskell formula is based on a decrease of 1 beat per year. The Tanaka formula is more accurate and reduces the risk that the patient will experience overexertion during stress testing. The Tanaka formula is as follows:

- 208 – (0.7 × age) = MHR
- 208 – (0.7 × 70) = 208 – 49 = 159

The Nes formula (2013) is designed for older adults that have higher than average fitness levels.

82. C: The radial and ulnar arteries are found in the wrist and are used when a practitioner is taking a pulse in a clinic. The popliteal artery is found in the leg posterior to the knee. The brachial artery is commonly palpated in the antecubital fossa, which is anterior to the elbow. The jugular artery is in the neck.

83. B: The J point is where the QRS complex transitions into the ST segment, marking where ventricular depolarization ends and repolarization begins. The J point may be on, above, or below the isoelectric line. Depression of the J point can be a normal finding, or it may indicate injury to the heart, hypokalemia, non–ST-segment elevation myocardial infarction, bundle branch block, or other cardiac abnormalities. Elevation of the J point can likewise be benign or may indicate cardiac injury, ST-segment elevation myocardial infarction, pericarditis, or Brugada syndrome.

84. D: An exercise stress test should be stopped immediately if the systolic BP is >250 mmHg or if the diastolic BP is >115 mmHg. The normal peak systolic BP ranges from 160–220 mmHg, although some patients can tolerate higher levels. An increase in systolic BP of less than 20 mmHg from baseline is abnormal. The systolic BP should decrease by 10–20 mmHg during the first minute of recovery. The diastolic BP usually remains stable or increases by 10 mmHg or less. It is uncommon for the diastolic BP to increase markedly during exercise.

85. D: A blood pressure cuff should ideally be placed on the upper arm, about half an inch above the elbow. The blood pressure cuff should be wrapped snugly around the arm in order to achieve proper compression of the brachial artery. You should be able to fit one finger underneath the cuff. If the cuff is too tight or too loose, the blood pressure reading may be inaccurate. Many cuffs have a brachial artery marker, which indicates how the cuff should be positioned on the arm (with the brachial artery marker just above the inner crease of the elbow).

86. D: Anyone who has taken a basic life support (BLS) course can do cardiopulmonary resuscitation (CPR). The BLS course involves a written examination and a simulation of maneuvers performed on a mannequin.

87. C: Underwire bras contain metal, which can conduct electrical signals, which can cause interference in the EKG signal. If the underwire is in contact with the electrodes, the resultant electrical circuit can lead to artifacts. The underwire may move during respirations, causing motion artifacts. The underwire can also pick up external electrical signals and cause AC interference (60 Hz), which can appear similar to a wandering baseline and may mask P waves, T waves, and ST segment changes.

88. C: The RL electrode in a 12-lead EKG serves as the ground electrode, which establishes a point of reference, or a baseline, for the EKG machine to interpret the signals from other electrodes. The RL electrode does not record the heart's electrical activity. The RL electrode helps filter out common electrical signals so that only the heart's electrical signals are detected. The RL electrode also helps reduce interference from muscle activity and improves the stability of the signal.

89. A: A sudden onset of slurred speech may be an indication of a stroke, an emergent situation, so the EKG technician should immediately call for help so that a healthcare professional, such as a nurse or physician, can assess the patient. There are two types of strokes:

- Ischemic (87%): Caused by plaque obstructing a vessel, a clot forming in an artery, or a clot traveling from another site to block an artery in the brain
- Hemorrhagic: Caused by rupture of a vessel and bleeding into the brain

90. C: The Osborn wave, also known as the J wave, on an EKG tracing is an upward deflection immediately after the R wave. The Osborn wave is found in patients who are hypothermic with temperatures of less than 35 °C (95 °F). The wave results from temperature-associated changes in the heart's electrical response, delaying ventricular repolarization. The size or amplitude of the wave increases as the body temperature decreases. The Osborn wave may also occur with hypercalcemia, sepsis, postresuscitation, and brain injury.

91. C: Breast implants consist of an outer shell of silicone elastomer and some type of filling material (e.g., saline, silicone gel, semisolid silicone gel, or silicone plus other material such as soy oil). Electrodes should never be placed over a breast implant because the implant will not conduct electrical activity, and this will interfere with signal transmission. Therefore, as with a normal female breast, the electrodes should be placed under the breast implants and as close as possible to the correct anatomical positions.

92. A, C, D: Because a stress test can place the patient at risk of an adverse cardiac event, the test should only be carried out if the proper equipment is readily available:

- Oxygen: Administered if oxygen saturation drops below 85% to relieve shortness of breath. Oxygen may also be used if the patient develops dizziness, arrhythmias, or chest pain.
- Automated external defibrillator/manual defibrillator: Used if cardiac arrest occurs to resuscitate the patient.
- Crash cart: Should contain life-saving medications (such as epinephrine and amiodarone), airway and respiratory equipment (e.g., endotracheal tubes, laryngoscope, bag-valve mask), and IV supplies.

93. C: The preferred method of hand-washing is the procedure in responses A or B. The procedure in response D is acceptable, but the use of antibacterial wipes is not.

94. C: The Lund lead system modification is done to reduce motion artifacts and is especially useful for patients such as those with Parkinson's disease or other causes of tremors. The Lund system may also be used with patients who are morbidly obese. With the Lund system, the limb leads are placed on the proximal areas of the limbs, the upper arms and the thighs, near the shoulders and hips. This has little or no effect on the waveforms, so this modification can be used for diagnostic EKGs.

95. C: Regardless of the size of a person's breasts or the person's gender, EKG electrodes should always be placed under the breast and never on top of the breast tissue to ensure EKG accuracy. Breast tissue is soft, so it can be more difficult to achieve a good electrode contact, and this tissue tends to move with respirations, which can result in increased artifacts. Placing the electrodes under the breast ensures correct placement along the rib cage.

96. D: With premature ventricular contractions (PVCs) and ventricular bigeminy, every normal beat is followed by a PVC. PVCs originate from an ectopic focus in the ventricles rather than from the SA node, so there is no P wave before a PVC. PVCs are characterized by a broad QRS complex (≥0.12 sec) with abnormal morphology. The PVC occurs earlier than expected. The T wave is negative if the QRS is positive, and it is positive if the QRS is negative.

97. D: During pregnancy, the blood volume increases by 40–60% and the cardiac output increases by 30–50%. In addition, the hormonal changes cause vasodilation and reduced BP. Combined, these changes result in a higher normal heart rate:

- First trimester: Increase of approximately 10 bpm
- Second trimester: Increase of approximately 15 bpm
- Third trimester: Increase of 15–20 bpm

Therefore, if the patient's baseline heart rate prior to becoming pregnant was 82 bpm, a heart rate of 100 (i.e., an increase of 18 bpm) is within the normal range.

98. D: A normal PR interval is 0.012–0.20 seconds on an EKG. Anything longer than 0.20 seconds is called a prolonged interval. Fixed, prolonged PR intervals are seen in first-degree heart block.

99. A: Pacemaker-mediated tachycardia can occur with dual- or triple-chamber implanted cardiac pacemakers that sense the atrium and pace the ventricle. The pacemaker mistakenly interprets retrograde conduction of P waves from the ventricles back to the atria and begins a reentrant loop of continuous pacing. On the EKG tracing, this appears as rapid pacemaker spikes before each QRS complex at a rate of <200 bpm (usually 120–150 bpm) with retrograde P waves evident following the QRS complex.

100. A: The underlying rhythm is a sinus rhythm. Premature atrial contractions (PACs) occur earlier than expected and originate outside of the SA node in another part of the atria. Because of this, the P wave has an abnormal appearance. There may be a compensatory pause after the PAC, but the QRS complex is usually normal—although, if the PAC occurs too early, it may not be conducted, and the QRS complex will be absent. PACs are usually benign and require no treatment if the patient is asymptomatic.

Answer Key and Explanations for Test #1

EKG Tech Practice Test #2

1. If a patient's heart rhythm is extremely irregular, the best method of calculating the heart rate is:

   a. Count the number of R-R intervals in 60 seconds.
   b. Count the QRS complexes in 6 seconds and multiply by 10.
   c. Count the number of small boxes between two consecutive R waves and divide by 1,500.
   d. Use the sequencing method (300, 150, 100, 75, etc.).

2. The following EKG tracing is characteristic of which electrolyte imbalance?

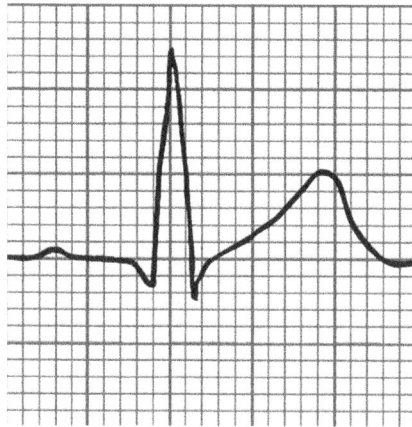

   a. Hyperkalemia
   b. Hypercalcemia
   c. Hypomagnesemia
   d. Hypermagnesemia

3. When reviewing a patient's list of drugs in order to be aware of any that may influence the EKG. When doing so, the EKG technician notes that the patient's list contains fentanyl patches. According to the drug schedule, how is fentanyl classified?

   a. Schedule I
   b. Schedule II
   c. Schedule III
   d. Schedule IV

4. After an impulse originates in the right upper atrium at the sinoatrial (SA) node, what does it travel through to get to the left atrium?

   a. Bachmann's bundle
   b. Bundle of His
   c. Purkinje fibers
   d. Left bundle branch

5. What is the name of the sounds heard during measurement of a manual blood pressure?

   a. Korsikoff.
   b. Kasakoff.
   c. Katankoff.
   d. Korotkoff.

6. If a patient has a demand pacemaker, the EKG technician would expect to see spikes on the EKG tracing:

 a. When the heart rate drops below a preset rate
 b. Only during atrial contraction
 c. At random intervals
 d. With every QRS complex

7. A patient's EKG strip indicates supraventricular tachycardia (SVT). Which of the following are characteristics of SVT? (Select the three [3] correct answers.)

 a. P wave absent, buried, or retrograde
 b. Heart rate of 120–200 bpm
 c. Heart rate of 150–250 bpm
 d. Sustained for long periods
 e. Paroxysmal in nature

8. Lead II on the EKG tracing measures the voltage between which two electrodes?

 a. Right arm and right leg
 b. Left leg and right arm
 c. Left leg and left arm
 d. Right leg and left arm

9. When using the R-R method to calculate the heart rate, what heart rate does this EKG strip represent?

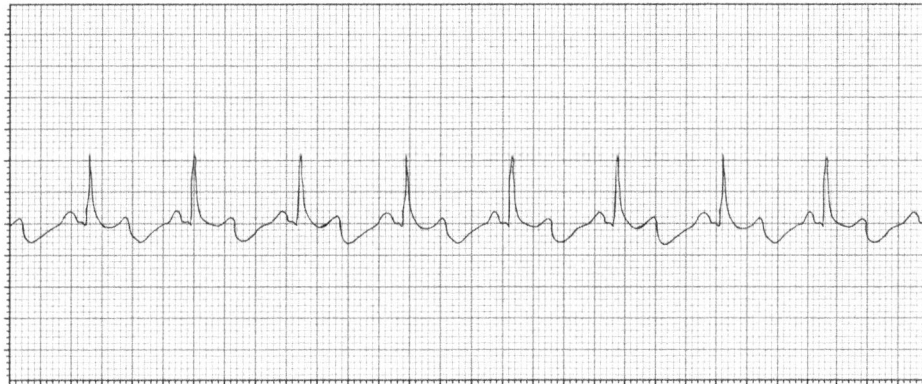

 a. 80
 b. 88
 c. 90
 d. 94

10. A heart rate of 125 beats per minute with absent or irregular p-waves best describes which of the following arrhythmias?

 a. Supraventricular tachycardia.
 b. Asystole.
 c. Atrial fibrillation.
 d. First-degree heart block.

11. When is the best time for a patient's blood pressure to be taken?

    a. While the patient is sleeping.
    b. While giving them unpleasant news.
    c. After sitting up in the bed or in a chair for several minutes.
    d. When getting undressed for an exam.

12. Which of the following pulse sites is normally used to take a pulse rate in emergencies?

    a. Radial pulse
    b. Brachial pulse
    c. Carotid pulse
    d. Apical pulse

13. Blood pressure is a function of all of the following EXCEPT:

    a. How strong the heart muscle is
    b. The elasticity of the arteries
    c. The size of the lumen of the arteries
    d. The ejection fraction

14. When communicating with a non-English speaking patient and her family, it is best to:

    a. Have another family member serve as an interpreter, if possible.
    b. Improvise using pictures and video to teach the patient about their medical care.
    c. Hold most of the conversation through an online translating program.
    d. Arrange to have an interpreter familiar with medical terminology present.

15. A patient has demonstrated the persistent rhythm shown on the following EKG tracing. What type of rhythm is this?

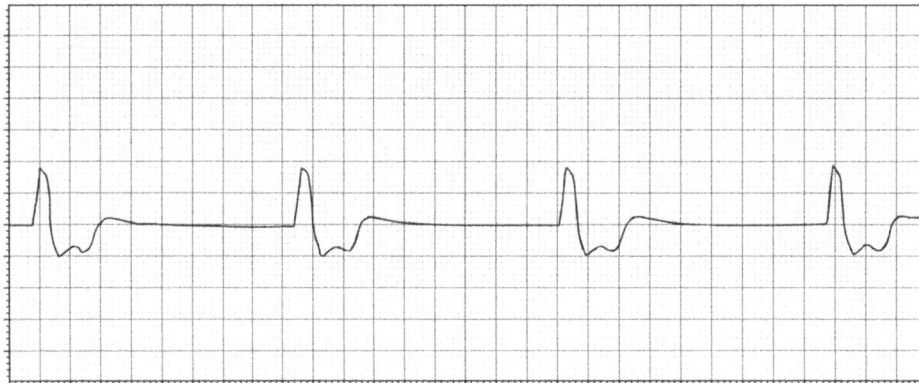

    a. Idioventricular rhythm
    b. Sinus bradycardia
    c. Agonal rhythm
    d. Complete (third-degree) heart block

16. If the duration of the QRS complex is 0.16 sec and the amplitude is 10 mm, how would these values be expressed in ms and mV?

    a. 1.6 ms and 1.0 mV
    b. 16 ms and 10 mV
    c. 160 ms and 10 mV
    d. 160 ms and 1.0 mV

17. If an error in an electronic medical record is discovered shortly after entry, how should it be corrected?

    a. Draw a single red line through the error, add the correction, indicate "Corr." or "Correction" above the error, and initial and date the area.

    b. Erase or white-out the error and put in the correct information.

    c. Set the computer software to track the error slot, line out the error with the dash key, make the correction to the right of the lined-out error, key in "Corr." or "Correction," and initial and date the error.

    d. Create a new citation identifying and correcting the error, sign and date it, and insert it into the original record.

18. Tachycardia in an adult is defined as a heart rate of:

    a. >120 bpm

    b. >110 bpm

    c. >100 bpm

    d. >90 bpm

19. An adult whose blood pressure is 125/85 is considered to have:

    a. Normal blood pressure

    b. Prehypertension

    c. Hypertension

    d. Secondary hypertension

20. If a patient who has been lying down stands up quickly and has a brief episode of syncope, the most likely cause is:

    a. Anxiety

    b. Vasovagal response

    c. Orthostatic hypotension

    d. Heart attack

21. How many electrodes are placed for a 12-lead EKG?

    a. 6

    b. 8

    c. 10

    d. 12

22. What is the normal duration of the P-R interval?

    a. 0.12–0.20 sec

    b. 0.18–0.24 sec

    c. <0.12 sec

    d. >0.24 sec

23. Prior to a pharmacologic stress test, patients should be advised to avoid all foods and liquids containing caffeine for at least:

    a. 4–6 hours

    b. 8–12 hours

    c. 12–18 hours

    d. 24 hours

24. Which of the following is a normal respiratory rate in a healthy adult?

   a. 6 breaths per minute.
   b. 16 breaths per minute.
   c. 26 breaths per minute.
   d. 36 breaths per minute.

25. Which of the following best describes the use of chemical germicidal agents on surfaces to kill most microorganisms?

   a. Sanitization
   b. Disinfection
   c. Sterilization
   d. Antisepsis

26. When applying sterile gloves or assisting in a sterile procedure, where should the hands and/or sterile objects be held?

   a. In front, at a distance from the body
   b. In front, at a distance from the body and above waist level
   c. Above waist level
   d. Toward the sterile field

27. What does the following EKG tracing represent?

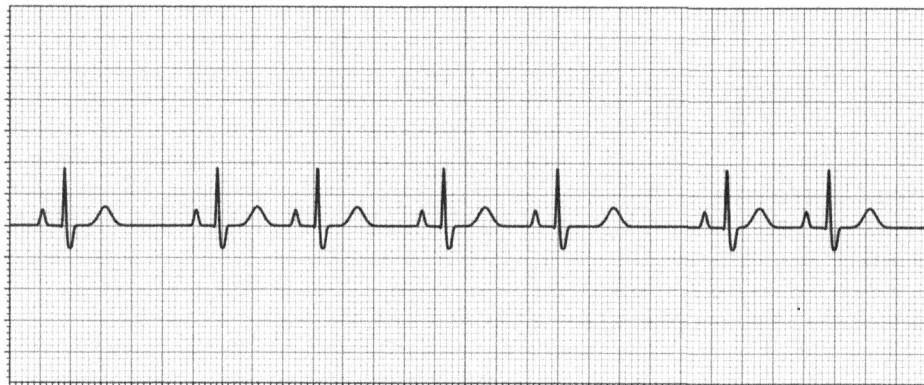

   a. Normal sinus rhythm
   b. Sinus arrhythmia
   c. First-degree AV block
   d. Second-degree AV block

28. On the waveform illustration below, to what does number 2 correspond?

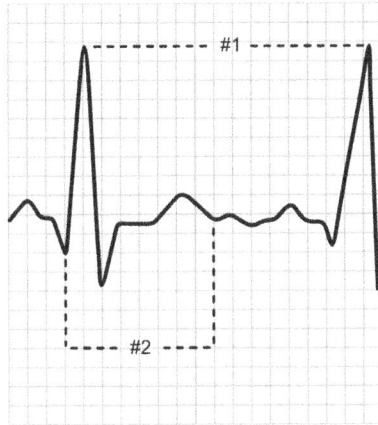

a. P-R interval
b. QT interval
c. ST segment
d. QRS complex

29. If an electrical current on an EKG is traveling perpendicular to the positive electrode, what type of deflection will occur?

a. Biphasic
b. Negative
c. Positive
d. None

30. What is the amplitude in millimeters of the T wave in the following EKG tracing?

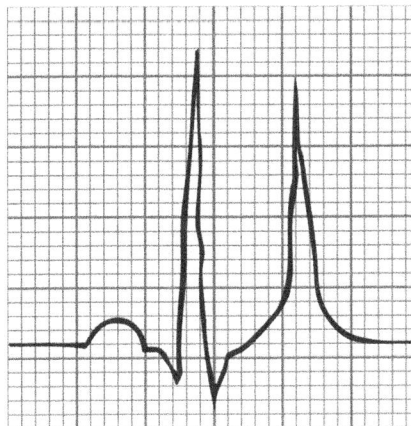

a. 5 mm
b. 4 mm
c. 3 mm
d. 2 mm

31. In the EKG strip below, what type of electrode misplacement is represented?

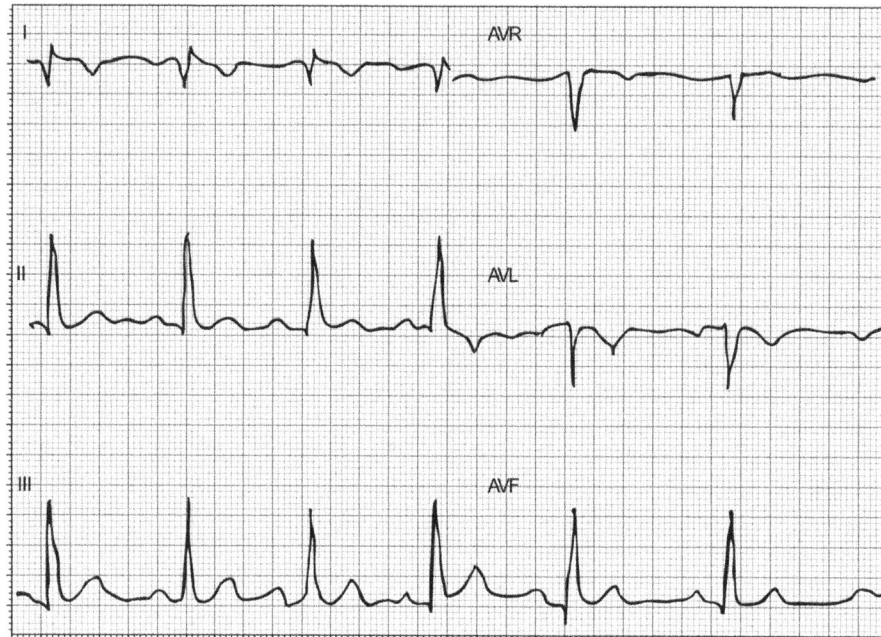

a. RA-LA
b. RL-LG
c. RA-RL
d. RA-LL

32. During an EKG, a patient appears cyanotic and apneic and the EKG technician cannot detect a palpable pulse. The EKG strip shows the following:

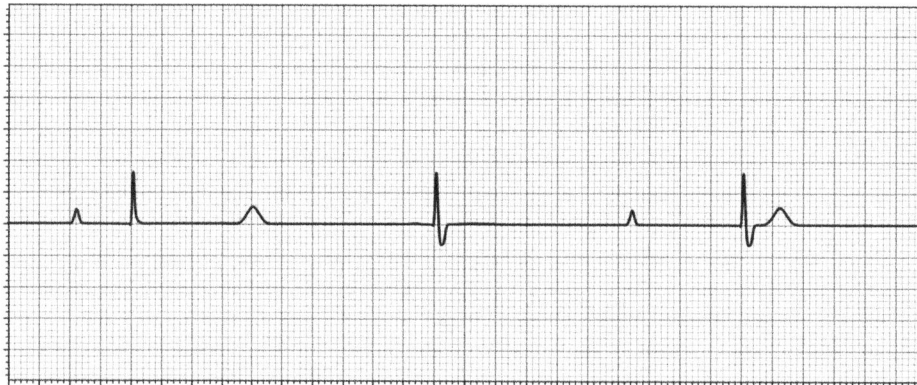

The EKG technician should suspect:
a. Pulseless electrical activity
b. Pulseless ventricular tachycardia
c. Normal sinus rhythm
d. Severe bradycardia

112

33. What piece of equipment is used for measuring blood pressure?

    a. Holter monitor.

    b. Sphygmomanometer.

    c. Urometer.

    d. Pulse oximeter.

34. For ambulatory event monitoring, what lead configuration is most commonly used?

    a. 3-lead

    b. 5-lead

    c. 7-lead

    d. 12-lead

35. Bradycardia in an adult is defined as a heart rate of:

    a. <80 bpm

    b. <70 bpm

    c. <60 bpm

    d. <50 bpm

36. What is the medical term for passing out?

    a. Tinnitus.

    b. Vertigo.

    c. Syncope.

    d. Hemiparesis.

37. Of the cardiac-related drugs that should be kept on hand in an ambulatory setting, which one is used for angina pectoris?

    a. Nitroglycerin

    b. Atropine

    c. Digoxin

    d. Isoproterenol

38. When is it appropriate to discuss a patient on social media?

    a. If their name is not disclosed.

    b. If their picture is not disclosed.

    c. If their diagnosis is not disclosed.

    d. It is never appropriate to discuss a patient on social media.

39. With a wandering atrial pacemaker, what part of the EKG wave is most altered?

    a. P wave

    b. P-R interval

    c. QRS complex

    d. T wave

40. Which of the following heart rhythms are potentially lethal? (Select the three [3] correct answers.)

    a. Atrial flutter
    b. Idioventricular rhythm
    c. VT
    d. Ventricular fibrillation
    e. Atrial fibrillation

41. What is the best statement that describes an emancipated minor?

    a. A person who is freed from control of their parents.
    b. Someone who is charged with a crime in their childhood.
    c. A person who is adopted in young adulthood.
    d. Someone who cannot make his or her own medical decisions.

42. If the maximum heart rate (MHR) using the Fox & Haskell formula is 148, how old is the patient?

    a. 62
    b. 68
    c. 72
    d. 76

43. A patient with paroxysmal supraventricular tachycardia (SVT) is to have mobile cardiac event monitoring for a 1-month period with three leads connected to a transmitter that sends a message to a cellphone that transmits EKGs to the company sponsoring the device. What is the maximum distance that the patient should be from the cellphone?

    a. 2 feet
    b. 4 feet
    c. 6 feet
    d. 10 feet

44. If setting up a patient for inpatient wireless telemetry, what EKG configuration is typically used?

    a. 3-lead
    b. 5-lead
    c. 7-lead
    d. 12-lead

45. Which of the following is not a sign of a myocardial infarction?

    a. Vision loss.
    b. Chest tightness.
    c. Shortness of breath.
    d. Jaw pain.

46. What is the correct placement for the V4 lead?

    a. Fourth intercostal space, left anterior axillary line
    b. Fourth intercostal space, left midclavicular line
    c. Fifth intercostal space, left midclavicular line
    d. Fifth intercostal space, left midaxillary line

47. What is the rhythm in the following EKG tracing?

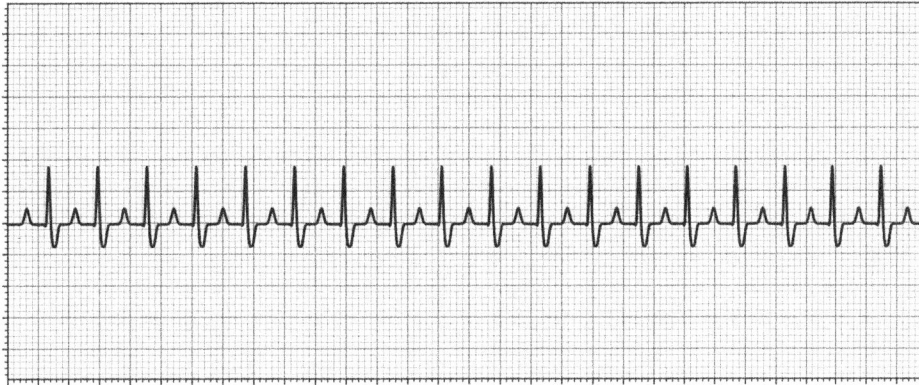

a. Normal sinus rhythm
b. Ventricular tachycardia
c. Atrial fibrillation
d. Atrial tachycardia

48. In a 12-lead EKG, how many precordial chest leads are there?

a. Two.
b. Four.
c. Six.
d. Eight.

49. What is the appropriate way to take a radial pulse?

a. Place your index finger and middle finger on the wrist, under the pinky finger
b. Place your index finger and middle finger on the wrist, under the thumb
c. Place your thumb on the side of the neck, next to the trachea
d. Place your index finger on the inner portion of the cubital fossa (anterior aspect of the elbow)

50. The rhythm on the following EKG tracing would be interpreted as:

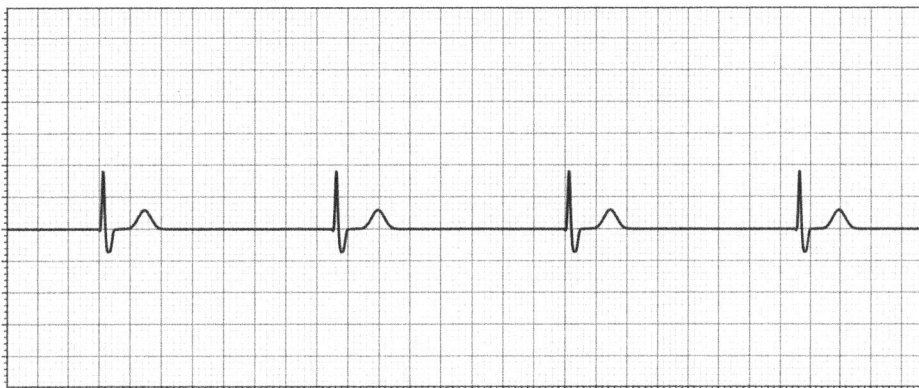

a. Sinus bradycardia
b. First-degree heart block
c. Junctional escape rhythm
d. Wandering atrial pacemaker

51. What type of sinoatrial (SA) block does the following EKG tracing demonstrate?

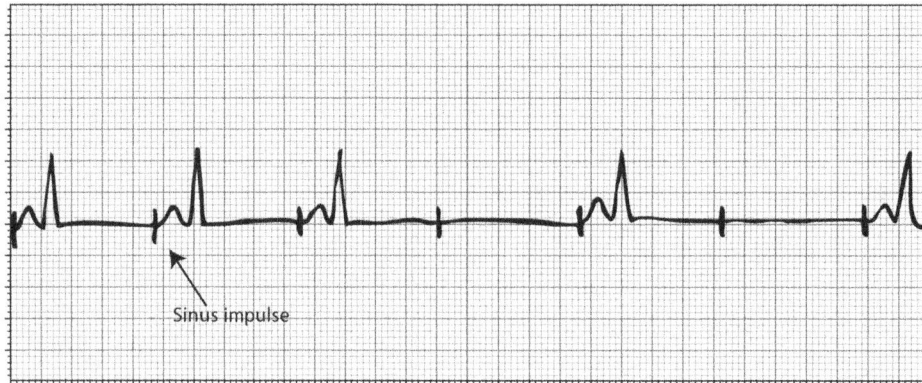

Sinus impulse

a. First-degree SA block
b. Second-degree SA block, type I
c. Second-degree SA block, type II
d. Third-degree SA block

52. If monitoring the oxygen saturation on a patient with very dark skin, the EKG technician should be aware that the skin color:

a. Has no effect on the readings
b. May result in falsely high readings
c. May result in falsely low readings
d. May result in falsely high or low readings

53. Following an exercise stress test, within the first minute, the heart rate recovery should be at least:

a. 30 bpm
b. 22 bpm
c. 12 bpm
d. 8 bpm

54. On an EKG strip recorded at 25 mm/sec, one large box on the *x*-axis is equal to:

a. 0.04 seconds
b. 0.10 seconds
c. 0.02 seconds
d. 0.20 seconds

55. Which of the following is not an appropriate method of communication to someone who is hearing impaired?

a. Hand gestures.
b. Pantomiming.
c. Speaking especially loudly.
d. Drawing pictures.

56. During which one of the following phases of the cardiac cycle do the coronary arteries fill with blood?

a. Atrial diastole
b. Atrial systole
c. Ventricular diastole
d. Ventricular systole

57. What is the duration of the P-R interval on the following EKG tracing?

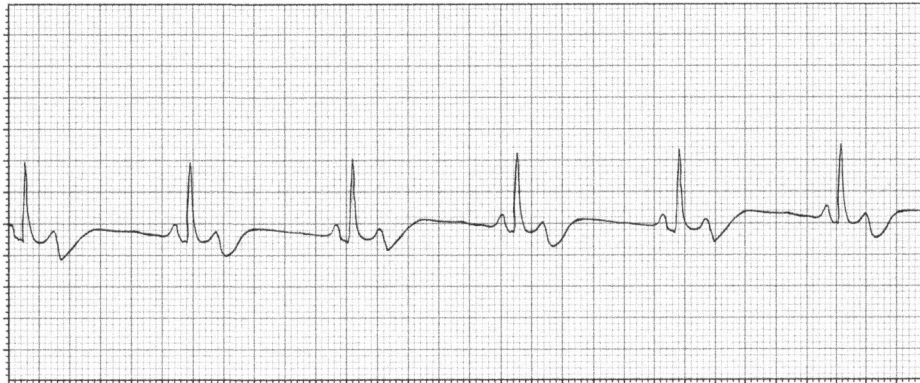

a. 0.10 sec
b. 0.12 sec
c. 0.14 sec
d. 0.16 sec

58. If the speed of an EKG is changed from 25 mm/sec to 50 mm/sec, how should the gain typically be adjusted?

a. No change is needed.
b. It should be decreased by half.
c. It should be increased by half.
d. It should be doubled.

59. Which formula for determining the maximum heart rate (MHR) is most accurate for the female physiology?

a. Fox & Haskell
b. Gellish
c. Gulati
d. Tanaka

60. In regard to the chain of infection, which would NOT be a portal of entry?

a. Ingestion.
b. Inhalation.
c. Perspiration.
d. Penetration.

61. If the normal respiratory rate is between 12 and 20 at rest, what is the anticipated respiratory rate at peak activity during an exercise stress test?

    a. 20–30
    b. 30–40
    c. 40–50
    d. 50–60

62. What is NOT a likely location for pulse oximeter placement?

    a. Fingertip.
    b. Sublingual.
    c. Earlobe.
    d. Toe.

63. If a physician suspects that a patient has had an inferior wall myocardial infarction and orders a posterior EKG with leads V7 through V9, these leads are placed on the back at the same level as:

    a. V1 and V2
    b. V3
    c. V4
    d. V6

64. If the waveform has the following appearance, what does this likely indicate?

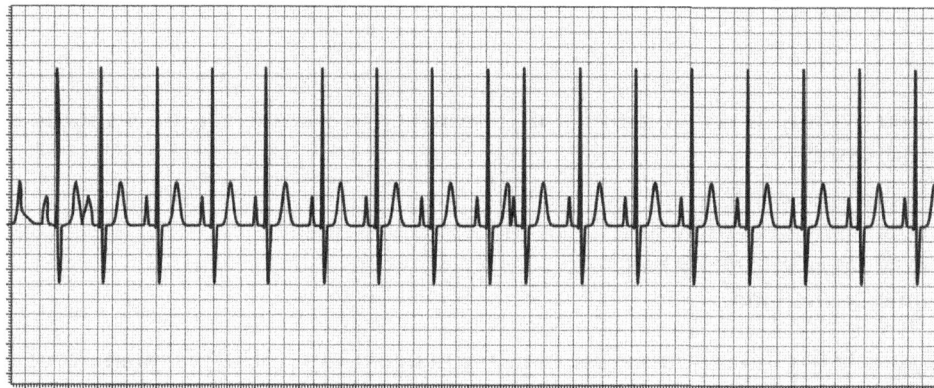

    a. Gain set too high
    b. SVT
    c. Electromagnetic interference
    d. Loose electrode

65. What does the EKG strip below indicate?

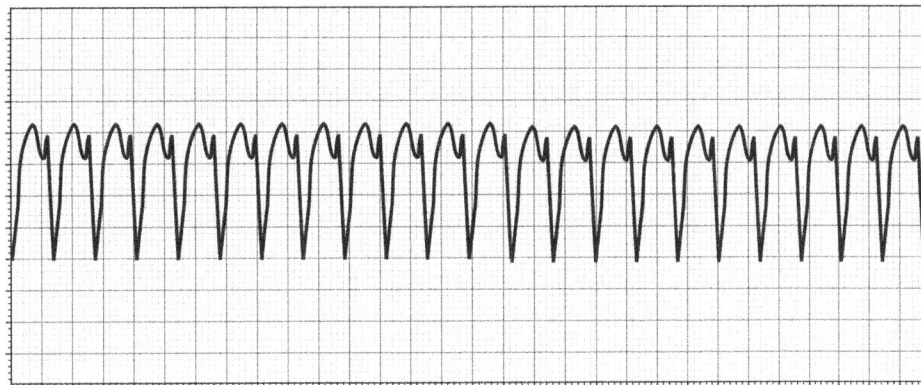

a. Ventricular paced rhythm
b. Supraventricular tachycardia
c. Atrial fibrillation
d. Ventricular tachycardia

66. What does the small positive deflection (indicated by the arrow) represent?

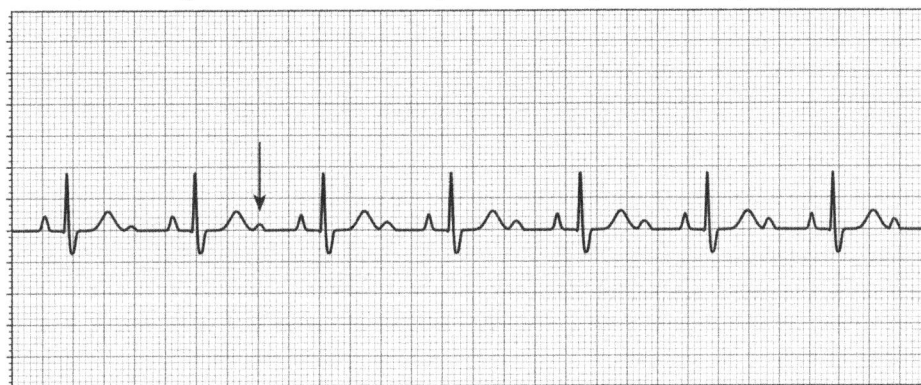

a. Notched T wave
b. Artifact
c. Premature P wave
d. U wave

67. When running a rhythm strip to check correct placement of limb electrodes, the EKG technician notes that lead III shows a negative QRST complex as well as a negative P wave. This suggests:

a. Reversal of the RL and RA electrodes
b. Reversal of the LA and LL electrodes
c. Reversal of the RL and LL electrodes
d. Reversal of the RA and LA electrodes

68. For the tilt-table test, the electrodes are generally placed while the patient is in:

a. Supine position
b. Low semi-Fowler's position
c. Trendelenburg
d. High semi-Fowler's position

69. **Which statement regarding the differences between surgical hand cleansing and medical hand cleansing is NOT true?**

    a. Surgical hand washing takes longer.
    b. During rinsing, hands should be down for medical hand cleansing and up for surgical hand cleansing.
    c. Lotion can be applied after medical hand cleansing, but not after surgical hand cleansing.
    d. Medical hand cleansing includes the forearm to the elbow, while surgical hand cleansing focuses only on the hands.

70. **Which of the following heart valves are semilunar? (Select the two [2] correct answers.)**

    a. Pulmonary
    b. Tricuspid
    c. Aortic
    d. Bicuspid

71. **The most common cause of excessive artifacts in an EKG tracing is:**

    a. Low battery
    b. Movement
    c. Electrical interference
    d. Improper electrode placement

72. **An irregular EKG, characterized by closely spaced premature ventricular contractions (PVCs), a lack of P waves, and distorted QRS complexes, indicates:**

    a. Atrial fibrillation
    b. Paroxysmal atrial tachycardia
    c. Ventricular tachycardia
    d. Ventricular fibrillation

73. **If a patient loses consciousness and the EKG tracing shows the following, the EKG technician should first:**

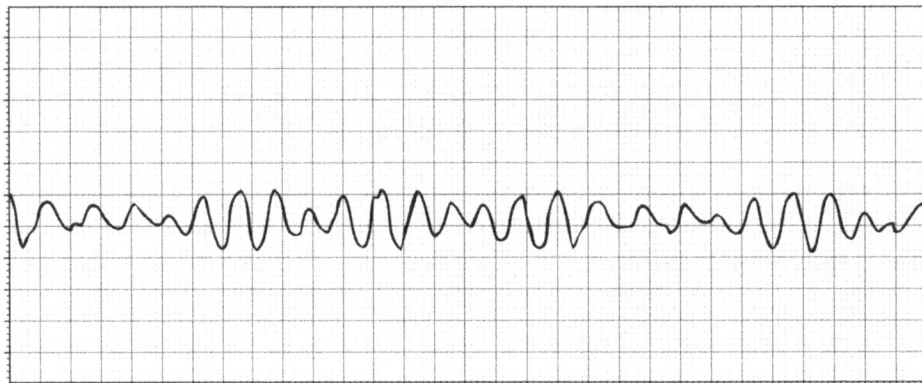

    a. Check the electrodes and leads.
    b. Print a strip for the healthcare provider.
    c. Attempt to arouse the patient.
    d. Call for help.

74. Which one of the following is an appropriate disinfectant to use to disinfect lead wires and EKG machine surfaces?

   a. Sodium hypochlorite >10% wipes
   b. Hydrogen peroxide 6% wipes
   c. 70% isopropyl alcohol wipes
   d. Ammonia-based wipes

75. Which leads are bipolar?

   a. I, II, III
   b. V1, V2, V3
   c. aVL, aVF, aVR
   d. V4, V5, V6

76. If a patient has a patch monitor, which of the following should be included in patient education? (Select the three [3] correct answers.)

   a. Avoid showering.
   b. Avoid tight-fitting clothes.
   c. Avoid placing an electric blanket over the patch.
   d. Avoid activities that cause excessive sweating.
   e. Avoid MRI scans.

77. If an adult patient collapses during a stress test, what is the correct site to check for a pulse for suspected cardiac arrest?

   a. Brachial artery
   b. Radial artery
   c. Temporal artery
   d. Carotid artery

78. Einthoven's triangle is formed by:

   a. Leads V4, V5, and V6
   b. Leads V1, V2, and V3
   c. Leads I, II, and III
   d. Any three leads

79. What is the primary purpose of a Holter monitor?

   a. Evaluate for vegetation.
   b. Diagnose heart attacks.
   c. Evaluate for arrhythmias.
   d. Determine ejection fraction.

80. What is the medical term for heart attack?

   a. Endocarditis.
   b. Pericardial effusion.
   c. Myocardial infarction.
   d. Myocarditis.

81. **The CDC guidelines for isolation of patients with highly transmissible diseases are to use:**
    a. Standard Precautions
    b. Personal protective equipment (PPE)
    c. Transmission-Based Precautions
    d. Standard Precautions and the applicable type of Transmission-Based Precautions

82. **The organization that works to ensure employee safety while performing job duties is:**
    a. Occupational Safety and Health Administration (OSHA)
    b. The Joint Commission
    c. The Americans with Disabilities Act
    d. The Food and Drug Administration (FDA)

83. **A patient who reports earlier chest pain but is now pain free, exhibits the following on an EKG tracing. These distinctive inverted T waves are referred to as:**

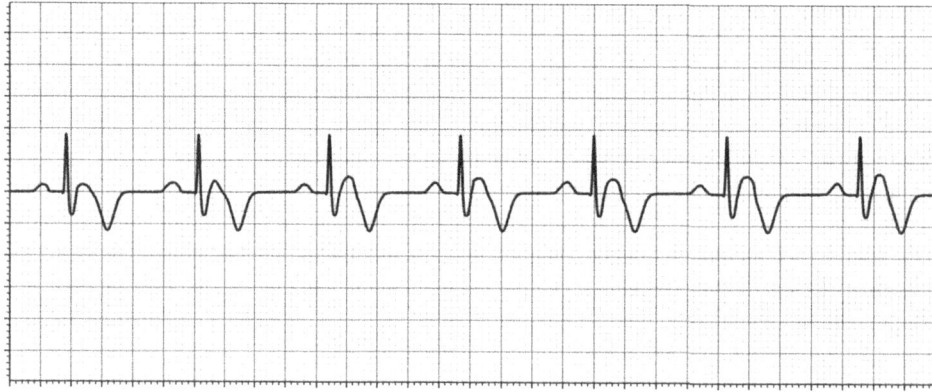

    a. De Winter's sign
    b. Camel-hump T waves
    c. Epsilon wave
    d. Wellens' syndrome

84. **If a patient has a Holter monitor (lead type), how long should he or she avoid taking a shower after its application?**
    a. For the entire duration of use
    b. For 12 hours
    c. For 24 hours
    d. For 48 hours

85. **The preferred method for disposal of sharps is to:**
    a. Use the scoop technique.
    b. Put them into a puncture-proof sharps container marked "biohazard."
    c. Put them in a metal pan for later sterilization.
    d. Recap the sharp and then put it in a sharps container.

86. **In an EKG tracing, which one of the following represents ventricular depolarization?**
    a. QRS complex
    b. ST segment
    c. PQR complex
    d. PQRST complex

87. If, under the US system, the right arm (RA) cable and electrode for the EKG is white, what color is used for the right arm cable and electrode for EKG equipment manufactured under the European system?

a. Yellow
b. Green
c. Red
d. Black

88. With three-lead EKG monitoring, the left arm electrode should be placed on the:

a. left lower arm
b. left upper arm
c. left upper torso
d. left lower torso

89. When preparing a patient for an exercise stress test, the EKG technician notes that the patient's oxygen saturation at rest is 86%. The EKG technician should:

a. Consult the healthcare provider
b. Ask the patient if he or she is feeling more shortness of breath than usual
c. Continue with the stress testing
d. Carry out the stress testing with oxygen

90. Using the Fox & Haskell model to determine the maximum heart rate and the Karvonen/heart rate reserve (HRR) method to determine the target heart rate for a 70-year-old patient with a resting heart rate of 82 and an exercise intensity of 50%, what is the target heart rate?

a. 116
b. 126
c. 136
d. 146

91. If a patient's heart rate had been running in the high 80s, but the sinoatrial (SA) node failed, and the atrioventricular (AV) node has taken over the pacing, what is the heart rate likely to be?

a. 60–80 bpm
b. 40–60 bpm
c. 20–40 bpm
d. 10–30 bpm

92. In the illustration below, what is the thorax line number 2 called?

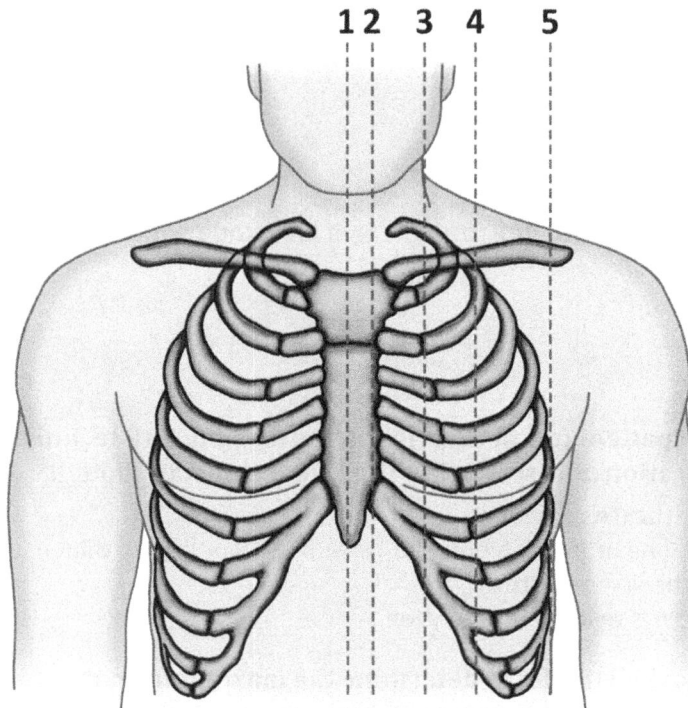

a. Midsternal line
b. Parasternal line
c. Sternal line
d. Midclavicular line

93. If a patient suffers from orthopnea, in what position should the patient be placed for a standard 12-lead EKG?

a. Supine, flat
b. Low semi-Fowler's (15–30 degrees)
c. Semi-Fowler's (30–45 degrees)
d. Full Fowler's (60–90 degrees)

94. The EKG technician is applying electrodes to prepare a patient for an exercise stress test, but the patient's chest is very hairy. The best solution is to:

a. Use clippers on areas of electrode placement.
b. Apply extra conducting gel.
c. Shave the areas of electrode placement.
d. Use a depilatory on areas of electrode placement.

95. If a pediatric patient is to have a 15-lead EKG, where is V4R placed?

a. Above the nipple at the right midclavicular line
b. Below the nipple at the right midclavicular line
c. On the left postaxillary line, level with V6
d. On the right postaxillary line, level with V3R

96. What would the waves occurring between the QRS complexes in the following EKG tracing be called?

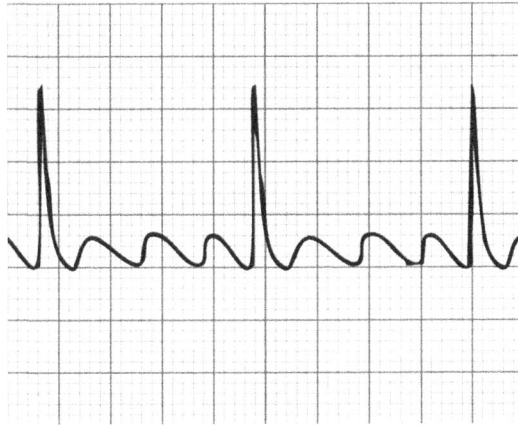

a. Flutter waves
b. Peaked T and W waves
c. Biphasic P wave
d. Biphasic T wave

97. What is the sequence for removing potentially contaminated personal protective equipment when exiting an isolation room?

a. Remove gown and gloves, remove goggles, remove mask, wash hands
b. Remove gown, remove goggles, remove mask, remove gloves, wash hands
c. Remove mask, remove goggles, remove gloves, remove gown
d. Remove gloves, wash hands, remove gown, remove mask

98. A patient must be monitored during a stress test for oxygen saturation with a pulse oximeter placed on an index finger. Which of the following may interfere with an accurate reading? (Select the three [3] correct answers.)

a. The patient has impaired circulation.
b. The patient's hands are very cold.
c. The patient has dry skin.
d. The patient has an elevated heart rate.
e. The patient is wearing black nail polish.

99. In the heart, blood is pumped from which chamber into the lungs?

a. Right atrium
b. Right ventricle
c. Left atrium
d. Left ventricle

100. An adult patient with trisomy 21 (Down syndrome) was accompanied in the waiting area by a parent and was quite calm, but once ushered toward the examination room, the patient becomes visibly agitated and frightened. The EKG technician should:

a. Reassure the patient.
b. Give the patient time to calm down.
c. Ask the patient what will help to relieve the anxiety.
d. Ask that the parent accompany the patient.

Answer Key and Explanations for Test #2

1. A: Although the 6-second method (i.e., counting the number of QRS complexes in a 6-second strip and multiplying by 10) is commonly used for an irregular rhythm, if a patient's heart rhythm is extremely irregular, determining an accurate heart rate can be challenging, and the 6-second strip is likely inadequate to make an accurate estimation. The most accurate method in this case is to count the number of R-R intervals in a 60-second EKG strip.

2. D: Hypermagnesemia (>2.5 mg/dL) can depress cardiac excitability and conduction, resulting in bradycardia, hypotension, heart block, and the risk of cardiac arrest, depending on the level of magnesium in the blood. Severe hypermagnesemia (>10 mg/dL) is a medical emergency because of the risk of cardiac arrest. Characteristic EKG findings of hypermagnesemia include a flattened P wave, a prolonged P-R interval (>0.20 sec), a widened QRS complex (>0.12 sec), a prolonged Q-T interval (>0.50 sec), and peaked T waves.

3. B: Fentanyl is a Schedule II drug. The Controlled Substances Act (1970) divides potentially addictive drugs into 5 different schedules:

- I. These are highly addictive substances with no medical use. Among them are heroin, ecstasy, marijuana (still classified as such, even though it has some medicinal uses), LSD, peyote, and bath salts (not the type for personal hygiene).
- II. These substances are highly addictive but have medicinal uses. Examples are fentanyl, morphine, demerol, codeine, Vicodin, and methadone.
- III. These substances pose a low to moderate risk of dependence or addiction. Among them are methadone, ketamine, anabolic steroids, and testosterone.
- IV. This schedule contains substances that pose a low risk of abuse/addiction. Examples are Xanax, Soma, Klonopin, Valium, and Ativan.
- V. These substances are the least addictive. Among them are cough suppressants like Robitussin AC and Ezogabine.

4. A: After an impulse originates in the right upper atrium at the sinoatrial (SA) node, it travels through Bachmann's bundle to the left atrium and down through the internodal tracts of the right atrium to the AV node and the bundle of His. From there, the electrical impulse travels to the right and left bundle branches and to the Purkinje fibers. Impulses travel more rapidly down the left bundle branch because the muscle is thicker. This allows both the right and left ventricles to contract at the same time.

5. D: The blood pressure cuff or sphygmomanometer and a stethoscope can be used to help measure blood pressure by auscultating Korotkoff sounds. Systolic pressure is registered as the pressure at which the sounds are first heard, and diastolic as the pressure at which they disappear.

6. A: A demand pacemaker discharges when the intrinsic heart rate falls below a preset rate, so pacemaker spikes will only appear on the EKG tracing when the pacemaker fires. This type of pacemaker is used most often for patients with episodes of intermittent bradycardia. A fixed-rate, or asynchronous, pacemaker fires at a constant rate, but this type is rarely used nowadays. Rate-responsive pacemakers adjust based on activity level. Single-chamber pacemakers pace only the atrium or ventricle, while dual-chamber pacemakers pace both chambers. Biventricular pacemakers pace both ventricles and sometimes also the atrium.

7. A, C, E: Supraventricular tachycardia (SVT) is a rapid heart rhythm that originates above the ventricles, such as in the atria or AV node. The heart rate is 150–250 bpm, and the P waves may be difficult or impossible to identify because they are absent, buried, or retrograde. The QRS complex is narrow and regular. SVT is typically paroxysmal in nature rather than sustained, so it begins and ends abruptly. SVT can be triggered by caffeine, stimulants, stress, or structural heart disease.

8. B: A lead in an EKG is a visual representation of the electrical activity of the voltage difference between two or more electrodes, with one electrode serving as the positive (+) pole and the other as the negative (–) pole. Lead I, for example, displays the voltage between the positive left arm electrode and the negative right arm electrode. Lead II on the EKG tracing displays the voltage between the positive left leg and negative right arm electrodes. Lead III displays the voltage between the positive left leg electrode and negative left arm electrodes.

9. B: There are 17 small boxes between the R waves. There are 1,500 small boxes in 1 minute; therefore, the formula is:

- 1,500/number of small boxes
- 1,500/17 = 88.2 = 88

The R-R method of determining the heart rate is most accurate with regular rhythms and is less accurate with irregular rhythms. The R-R method is simple and can be completed rapidly.

10. C: Atrial fibrillation is the abnormal arrhythmia where the atria do not rhythmically contract. This can cause palpitations, chest pain, dizziness, and syncope. It can result in pulmonary emboli, heart attack, and stroke. On an EKG the p-waves are irregular and not associated with QRS complexes.

11. C: A blood pressure should be taken once a patient has been seated or lying down for several minutes. If it is taken after an activity, it may be falsely elevated.

12. C: During emergency situations, the pulse site used is normally the carotid pulse, which is located on either side of the front of the neck, between the larynx and sternocleidomastoid muscle. In other situations, the radial pulse above the base of the thumb on the wrist, and the brachial pulse in the antecubital space on the inner side of the elbow, are commonly used sites. The apical pulse is located at the apex of the heart, can only be found using a stethoscope, and is typically used only in cardiac patients or infants. Other pulse sites include the temporal, femoral, popliteal, and dorsalis pedis artery sites.

13. D: Blood pressure is a function of how strong the heart muscle is and the elasticity of the arteries, as well as blood volume and blood viscosity. The size of the lumen of the arteries is directly related to their peripheral resistance, which also impacts blood pressure. Ejection fraction represents the volume of blood that is released from the heart with every contraction, but does not directly affect blood pressure.

14. D: Whenever possible, have an interpreter present in these types of situations, ideally one who has undergone some training in medical terminology. Using a family member is not ideal because it is not known if they are able to translate medical terms correctly. Online software may not be accurate and there is no way to verify that the terms and concepts are being interpreted appropriately. Pictures and videos will enhance communication provided through an interpreter.

15. A: Idioventricular rhythm occurs when the SA and AV nodes are not sending signals at a high enough rate, so the ventricle's myocardium serves as the pacemaker, but, since the intrinsic rate of the ventricles is only 20–40 bpm, the heart rate is slow although the rhythm is regular. The P wave and the P-R interval are absent, and the QRS complex is typically wide (>0.10 sec) and may be bizarrely shaped.

16. D: To convert seconds (sec) to milliseconds (ms), multiply the sec by 1,000 (or move the decimal point three places to the right):

- $0.16 \times 1,000 = 160$ ms

To convert millimeters (mm) to millivolts (mV), remember that 10 mm = 1 mV, so divide the number of mm by 10:

- 10 mm/10 = 1.0 mV

When reporting EKG values, mm is used more frequently than mV, and sec is used more often than ms.

17. C: When using an electronic medical record, this is the way of correcting errors discovered promptly. Response D describes how to make these corrections later, after the software locks out the method in response C. Responses A and B describe right and wrong ways, respectively, to make corrections on paper medical records.

18. C: Tachycardia in an adult is defined as a heart rate of >100 bpm (usually 100–180). The most common type is sinus tachycardia, in which the rate is rapid but regular. The rhythm is regular, and the P wave morphology is upright in leads I, II, and aVF and inverted in aVR. The P-R interval and QRS complex are normal. However, the T wave may be somewhat flattened because of the rapid heart rate, and the Q-T interval may be shortened.

19. B: An adult with this blood pressure (BP) reading is considered to have prehypertension, which can lead to hypertension if not controlled. Normal blood pressure for an adult is a systolic pressure less than 120 and a diastolic pressure less than 80. Any BP above 140/90 is considered hypertension. Secondary hypertension is high blood pressure due to some underlying cause, such as atherosclerosis. If atherosclerosis is treated, the BP can return to normal or close to normal.

20. C: Gravity pulls the blood downward when a person stands. The autonomic nervous system compensates by increasing the heart rate and constricting blood vessels. If this system fails or the response is delayed, it can result in orthostatic hypotension. Orthostatic hypotension occurs when a person stands up and experiences a systolic BP drop of ≥20 mm Hg or a diastolic BP drop of ≥10 mm Hg. This usually happens immediately, but it can occur within 3 minutes, so patients should be advised to get up slowly and take deep breaths before walking, especially patients who are ill or elderly.

21. C: The 12-lead EKG requires 10 electrodes:

Limb electrodes (four electrodes)

- RA (right arm)—white: Right wrist or shoulder
- LA (left arm)—black: Left wrist or shoulder
- RL (right leg)—green: Right ankle or lower abdomen (serves as a ground)
- LL (left leg)—red: Left ankle or lower abdomen

Chest (precordial) electrodes (six electrodes)

- V1—Fourth intercostal space, right of the sternum
- V2—Fourth intercostal space, left of the sternum
- V3—Midway between V2 and V4
- V4—Fifth intercostal space, midclavicular line
- V5—Fifth intercostal space, anterior axillary line
- V6—Fifth intercostal space, midaxillary line

22. A: The normal duration of the P-R interval is 0.12–0.20 sec (3–5 small boxes). The P-R interval is the time needed for the electrical impulse to go from the sinoatrial (SA) node through the atrioventricular (AV) node to the ventricles. A shortened P-R interval occurs when conduction is accelerated, such as with Wolff-Parkinson-White syndrome. A prolonged P-R interval is indicative of AV block, which, if untreated, can progress to heart failure or bradycardia.

23. D: Caffeine is a stimulant that can increase the heart rate, blood pressure (BP), and cardiac workload, which can lead to false-positive results for the stress test. Additionally, it the patient is scheduled for a pharmacologic stress test, caffeine can block the effects of adenosine. Patients are advised to avoid food and drinks containing caffeine for 12–24 hours prior to an exercise stress test; however, patients scheduled for a pharmacologic stress test should avoid caffeine for 24 hours.

24. B: A normal respiratory rate in a healthy adult is 12–20 breaths per minute. Below this range is called bradypnea, and above this range is called tachypnea.

25. B: The use of chemical germicidal agents on surfaces by wiping or soaking is known as disinfection; it destroys most pathogens, but not spores. Sanitization is the use of techniques such as enzymatic detergents and ultrasonic cleaners to reduce microbial load on instruments and equipment. Sterilization is the use of techniques such as steam sterilization to kill all microbes, including spores. Antisepsis is the use of topical chemicals on the skin to kill or inhibit microbes.

26. B: In order to maintain sterility, both hands should be held in front of the body, at a distance from the body, and above waist level.

27. B: Sinus arrhythmia is characterized by irregular R-R intervals but with normal P waves preceding every QRS complex. Typically, this is a normal variation caused by changes in respirations. The R-R interval decreases with inspiration and increases during expiration. Sinus arrhythmia is most common in children, young adults, and athletes. Older adults may exhibit nonrespiratory sinus arrhythmia because of sick sinus syndrome, sinus node dysfunction, or use of some medications, such as beta blockers and digoxin.

28. B: On the illustration, number 2 represents the QT interval, which starts at the beginning of the Q wave and continues until the end of the T wave. The QT interval represents ventricular depolarization (QRS complex) and ventricular repolarization (ST segment and T wave). The normal QT interval is <440 ms in males and <460 ms in females. A prolonged QT interval is a risk for a ventricular arrhythmia (torsades de pointes), and a shortened QT interval may indicate a metabolic abnormality such as hypercalcemia.

29. A: If an electrical current moves toward the positive electrode, the deflection is positive, such as the P wave, T wave, and QRS complex in lead II (RA to LL). If the current moves away from the positive electrode, the deflection is negative or inverted, such as in lead aVR where the heart's electrical activity moves away from the positive RA electrode. With lead V3, the electrical current moves perpendicular to it, resulting in a biphasic waveform with part of the wave being positive and part being negative, such as the P wave, QRS, or T wave in V3 and V4.

30. B: To measure the amplitude of a wave, measure from the baseline to the peak or trough of the wave, depending on whether the deflection is positive or negative. In this case, the peak of the T wave is four small boxes above the baseline. Each small box represents 1 mm, so the amplitude of the T wave is 4 mm, or 0.4 mV. The normal amplitude of the T wave varies from ≤5 mm in limb leads to ≤10 mm in precordial leads. The normal T wave duration is 0.10–0.25 sec.

31. A: This EKG strip is typical of right arm/left arm (RA-LA) lead misplacement:

- Lead I shows inversion (negative deflection) of the P wave and the QRS complex because of reversed polarity.
- Leads II and III switch appearances.
- Leads aVR and aVL reverse so that aVR, which is normally negative, becomes positive and aVL, which is normally positive, becomes negative.
- The rhythm is unchanged since there is no major effect on AVF, VI–V6.

32. A: With elect electrical activity, some type of cardiac electrical activity is present but no mechanical activity or contractions are taking place, so there is no palpable pulse and the heart cannot maintain systemic perfusion. Its appearance on the EKG may vary. For example, it may present as a normal sinus rhythm. The EKG technician should call for help and begin CPR. Pulseless electrical activity does not respond to defibrillation but is treated with epinephrine.

33. B: The blood pressure cuff or sphygmomanometer and a stethoscope can be used to help measure blood pressure by auscultating Korotkoff sounds. Systolic pressure is registered as the pressure at which the sounds are first heard, and diastolic as the pressure at which they disappear.

34. A: Ambulatory event EKG monitoring is used to record the electrical activity of the heart for extended periods, so it is important that the electrodes do not limit mobility. Event recorders are especially useful for patients who have infrequent episodes or who are unaware of any symptoms. They may also be used to monitor the effects of medications or an implanted pacemaker. Typically, the 3-lead configuration is used:

- RA: Right chest, below the clavicle
- LA: Left chest below the clavicle
- LL: Lower left chest or upper abdomen

35. C: Bradycardia in an adult is defined as a heart rate of <60 bpm. Sinus bradycardia is the most common type in which the sinus node generates impulses at a slower than normal rate. This slow rate is common in athletes, during sleep, and with vasovagal syndrome. The rhythm is regular, and the P wave morphology is upright in leads I, II, and aVF and is inverted in aVR. The P-R interval, QRS complex, and T wave are normal, although the Q-T interval may be prolonged because of the slow heart rate.

36. C: Syncope is the medical term for passing out. There are many etiologies that may cause syncope, such as stress, hemorrhage, hypoglycemia, bradycardia, pregnancy, vertigo, stroke, and hypoxia.

37. A: Nitroglycerin, a vasodilator, is used to treat an attack of angina pectoris or chest pain due to chronic heart disease. Atropine is used to increase heart rate. Digoxin is used in congestive heart failure or arrhythmias. Isoproterenol is used to treat heart blocks. Other types of drugs should also be available, such as albuterol (bronchodilator), epinephrine (vasoconstrictor for anaphylactic shock), and prochlorperazine (an antiemetic).

38. D: Discussing a patient or any aspect of their case on social media is a violation of HIPAA. HIPAA requires that all employees of a medical facility maintain patient confidentiality.

39. A: With a wandering atrial pacemaker, the electrical impulse shifts from the SA node to other areas of the atria and to the AV junction, resulting in at least three different P wave morphologies (leads II, III, aVF):

- SA node: Normal in appearance.
- Near the SA node: Normal or slightly prolonged.
- Midatrial area: May be biphasic, the P-R interval may be slightly shorter than normal.
- Near AV node: Inverted because the impulse is retrograde, and the P-R interval is shorter than normal.
- AV junction: Inverted; the P-R interval is very short, and the wave may be buried in the QRS complex.

40. B, C, D: Potentially lethal heart rhythms:

- Idioventricular rhythm can become an agonal rhythm if it is sustained because it depends on the intrinsic rate of the Purkinje fibers; however, since this is only 20–40 bpm, it may not be enough to sustain life.
- VT may become pulseless or unstable and deteriorate into ventricular fibrillation. If pulseless, defibrillation is required. If unstable, cardioversion is required.
- Ventricular fibrillation results in disorganized electrical activity and requires immediate defibrillation.

41. A: An emancipated minor is a person younger than 18 who has been freed from control of his or her parents. He or she must provide for themselves financially, and his or her parents are not legally responsible for the child's actions.

42. C: The maximum heart rate (MHR) is the highest rate the body can achieve at maximum effort. The Fox & Haskell formula is commonly used for general fitness because it is easy to calculate. However, because there is considerable individual variability, this formula should be used only as a general guideline. With the Fox & Haskell formula, the person's age is subtracted from 220:

- 220 – age = MHR

If the MHR is 148, the age is calculated by subtracting 148 from 220:

- 220 – 148 (MHR) = 72 (patient's age).

43. D: If a patient with paroxysmal supraventricular tachycardia (SVT) is to have mobile cardiac event monitoring for a 1-month period with three leads connected to a transmitter that sends a message to a cellphone that transmits EKGs to the company, the maximum distance that the patient should be from the cellphone is 10 feet; therefore, the patient should attach the transmitter and the cellphone to his or her waist or carry the cellphone in a pocket or purse.

44. A: For inpatient wireless telemetry, a 3-lead EKG configuration is typically used because it allows for monitoring of noncritical cardiac arrhythmias while not unduly restricting patient mobility. The 3-lead configuration can detect atrial fibrillation, bradycardia, tachycardia, and pauses, but it is less effective for detection of ST-segment changes; therefore, the 12-lead system is more useful for diagnostic purposes. The 3-lead system is relatively inexpensive compared to 5- to 12-lead systems and requires less time to set up.

45. A: Vision loss is not a sign of a heart attack (myocardial infarction). A heart attack occurs when the cardiac cells in a portion of the heart die due to prolonged insufficient blood and oxygen flow. Signs and symptoms may include chest pain, shortness of breath, jaw pain, palpitations, diaphoresis, nausea, vomiting, dizziness, and feeling of impending doom.

46. C: Chest leads must be correctly placed because incorrect placement can alter waveforms and lead to incorrect interpretation. Chest-lead placement for a 12-lead EKG:

- Lead V1: fourth intercostal space, to the right of the sternum
- Lead V2: fourth intercostal space, to the left of the sternum
- Lead V3: Between leads V2 and V4
- Lead V4: Fifth intercostal space, left midclavicular line
- Lead V5: Fifth intercostal space, anterior axillary line
- Lead V6: Fifth intercostal space, midaxillary line

47. D: With atrial tachycardia, a type of SVT, electrical impulses are generated from a single area of the right or left atrium at a rate that is so rapid that it overrides the SA node. On the EKG, atrial tachycardia is characterized by a rapid atrial rate (100–250 bpm). P waves are typically abnormal in shape or may be hidden in the preceding T wave. The rhythm is regular, and the QRS complex is normal.

48. C: To obtain a 12-lead EKG, a total of 10 electrodes are used. Six precordial chest leads and four limb leads are used.

49. B: The radial pulse is palpated at the wrist, under the thumb. When taking a pulse, you should use the pads of your index finger and middle finger. Your thumb has a pulse beat of its own, which may interfere with feeling the patient's pulse. The carotid pulse is palpated on the side of the neck, next to the trachea. The brachial pulse is palpated on the inner portion of the cubital fossa (anterior aspect of the elbow). The ulnar artery pulse is located at the wrist, under the pinky, but it is not as commonly used as the radial pulse.

50. C: Junctional escape rhythm occurs when the SA node fails to generate electrical impulses or the impulses are blocked so that the AV node takes over as the pacemaker. This results in retrograde depolarization, which affects the P wave and the P-R interval. The P wave and the P-R interval are often absent, but the P wave may be inverted or retrograde (after the QRS complex). The heart rate with junctional escape rhythm is usually 40–60 bpm.

51. B: With a sinoatrial (SA) block, there is a conduction delay or failure of impulse transmission from the SA node to the atria, resulting in intermittent pauses in the heart rhythm. First-degree SA block is not observable on an EKG because the SA conduction delay still reaches the atria. This is an example of second-degree SA block, type I (Wenckebach). There is a progressive shortening of the P-P interval that occurs before a dropped beat as the electrical impulse progressively weakens before failing.

52. B: The pulse oximeter may register falsely high readings on a patient with dark skin because the it measures how much red and infrared light is absorbed by oxygenated versus deoxygenated hemoglobin. The melanin in dark skin increases the absorption of light. Thus, patients with dark skin must be monitored carefully for signs of respiratory distress and should be advised to indicate any increased shortness of breath because they are at risk for undetected hypoxia.

53. C: The heart rate recovery after exercise is the rate at which the heart slows. This is closely monitored for at least the first 3 minutes or until the patient returns to baseline:

- Heart rate recovery 1 minute: ≥12 bpm
- Heart rate recovery 2 minutes: ≥22 bpm
- Heart rate recovery 3 minutes: >30 bpm

If the heart rate recovery is faster than normal, this is typically an indication of good cardiovascular fitness. If the heart rate recovery is slower than normal, this can indicate autonomic dysfunction, poor physical fitness, a higher resting heart rate, chronic heart disease, or the use of beta blockers or other medications that lower the heart rate.

54. D: On an EKG strip recorded at 25 mm/s, one large box is equal to 0.20 seconds and each small box is equal to 0.04 seconds. The x-, or horizontal, axis measures time, while the y-, or vertical, axis measures amplitude or voltage. If a heart rate is very rapid, a recording rate of 50 mm/s may provide a better visualization of the waveform.

Measure	25 mm/s	50 mm/s
Small square	0.04 sec	0.02 sec
Large square	0.20 sec	0.10 sec

55. C: Speaking especially loud or yelling to a person who may not be able to hear is not appropriate. An alternative way of communicating may include hand gestures, pantomiming, writing out questions, or drawing pictures.

56. C: Ventricular diastole. Cardiac cycle:

9. Atrial systole: The atria contract, pushing blood into the ventricles. The tricuspid and mitral valves are open, and the pulmonary and aortic valves are closed.
10. Atrial diastole: The atria relax and fill with blood from the superior vena cava and the pulmonary veins. The tricuspid and mitral valves remain open, and the pulmonary and aortic valves remain closed.
11. Ventricular systole: The ventricles contract and eject blood. The tricuspid and mitral valves close, and the pulmonary and aortic valves open.
12. Ventricular diastole: The ventricles relax and fill. The tricuspid and mitral valves open, and the pulmonary and aortic valves close. Blood fills the coronary arteries.

57. D: The following is an example of sinus bradycardia. The P-R interval is 0.16 sec (four small boxes × 0.04), which is within the normal range of 0.12–0.20 sec. The heart rate is regular at approximately 43 bpm (seven large boxes), and the P waves are present and upright with one P wave present before each QRS segment. The QRS complex is 0.08 sec, so it is within the normal range (0.06–0.10 sec).

58. A: If the speed of an EKG is changed from 25 mm/s to 50 mm/s, the gain typically does not need to be adjusted. The purpose of changing the speed is to expand the waveform so it is easier to interpret, such as with an infant with a very rapid heart rate. However, the gain measures the height or amplitude of the waveform, and the change in speed does not affect the amplitude; therefore, it does not need to be changed. The amplitude is typically set as 10 mm/mV, which should produce a 10 mm deflection.

59. C: The Gulati formula, developed by Martha Gulati, MD (2010), was designed specifically for women because women normally have lower MHR values than men of the same age. Therefore, some formulas, such as the Fox & Haskell formula, overestimate the MHR for women. The Gulati formula is as follows:

- $206 - (0.88 \times age) = MHR$

For example, if a woman is age 60:

- $206 - (0.88 \times 60) = 206 - 52.8 = 153.2 = 153$ (MHR)

Using the Fox & Haskell formula for a woman of the same age would calculate her MHR to be 160.

60. C: There are three portals of entry for an infection to spread: ingestion (fecal-oral transmission), inhalation (respiratory droplet), and penetration (sexually transmitted disease). Infections are not transmitted through sweating.

61. B: The normal respiratory rate at rest is 12–20; however, at peak exercise, the anticipated respiratory rate should be between 30 and 40 for most individuals. At maximal exercise, the respiratory rate may increase further, but this degree of effort should not be evident with an exercise stress test. The respiratory rate increases because the muscles need more oxygen. Rapid, shallow breathing may occur with lung disease. An increase of greater than 50 bpm early in the test can indicate poor cardiovascular fitness, inefficient ventilation, or anxiety. A blunted rate may indicate heart failure, neuromuscular disease, or obesity hypoventilation syndrome.

62. B: A pulse oximeter is a medical device that indirectly monitors the oxygen saturation of a patient's blood. It is usually placed on a peripheral body part. The fingertip is most commonly used but can also be placed on a toe or an earlobe.

63. D: Posterior EKGs are used to detect posterior wall myocardial infarctions and inferior or lateral ST-elevation myocardial infarctions. With a posterior EKG, the electrodes for leads V7 through V9 are placed on the back at the same level as V6, at the fifth intercostal space. While leads V1 through V3 are left in standard positions, the lead wires for V4, V5, and V6 are typically used for V7, V8, and V9 with V7 on the back at the midaxillary line, V8 at the midscapular line, and V9 at the midline.

64. A: This likely indicates that the gain is set too high and should be checked. Gain measures the amplitude of the EKG signal, and most EKG machines are set by default at 10 mm/mV, meaning that a 1 mV electrical signal will produce a 10 mm deflection. If the gain is set too high, the QRS complex may appear very large, suggesting hypertrophy, and some overlapping of the P and T waves may make the EKG hard to interpret. EKG machines can be adjusted to make the waveform higher (20 mm) or lower (5 mm).

65. D: With ventricular tachycardia (VT), there is reduced cardiac output because the rapid ventricular contractions are inefficient. VT can progress to ventricular fibrillation and cardiac arrest; therefore, VT represents an emergent condition. VT is characterized by:

- Rapid ventricular rate (100–250 bpm).
- Wide QRS complexes (≥230 milliseconds [ms]/three small boxes)
- Absent or dissociated P waves
- Consistent shape and duration of QRS complexes OR changes in shape, amplitude, and direction
- Generally, a regularly spaced R-R interval

66. D: The U wave is the small positive deflection (best observed in leads V2 and V3) that is believed to represent repolarization of the Purkinje fibers, although the U wave is not completely understood. The U wave is most commonly observed in patients with a heart rate of 65 or lower and is generally a normal finding. A prominent U wave can be an indication of hypokalemia or hypercalcemia, but it is also found in athletes. Inverted U waves may be an indication of hypertension or acute ischemia.

67. B: If a rhythm strip shows a negative QRST complex as well as a negative P wave in lead III, the EKG technician should suspect a reversal of the LA and LL electrodes. Lead III measure the electrical potential difference between the LA and LL electrodes. The LL electrode is positive, and the LA is negative and produces positive deflections in lead III. Reversing the LA and LL electrodes alters the polarity of lead III, resulting in negative deflections instead of positive.

68. A: The tilt-table test assesses patients with unexplained episodes of light-headedness or syncope. The patient's EKG and vital signs are continuously monitored to assess changes in heart rhythm and BP in relation to changes in posture. The electrodes are applied with the patient lying flat in supine position, and a baseline recording is obtained. The head of the table is gradually tilted to 60–80 degrees. The patient remains in this position for 20–45 minutes and then returns to horizontal. If no symptoms occur, the patient may be given a medication, such as nitroglycerine, to provoke a response.

69. D: Surgical hand cleansing extends to the elbows, while medical hand cleansing is focused on the hands. Surgical hand washing takes longer and hands are held up during rinsing. Hands are held down during medical hand cleansing, and lotion can be applied after. Additional differences include that alcohol-based products can be substituted for medical washing but are only used after other steps in surgical washing, and that gloves are always applied after surgical hand cleansing.

70. A, C: There are two different classifications of heart valves. The semilunar valves are located between the ventricles and arteries, while the AV valves are located between the atria and the ventricles. AV valves include the tricuspid valve between the right atrium and right ventricle and the bicuspid (mitral) valve between the left atrium and left ventricle. The semilunar valves include the pulmonary valve between the right ventricle and pulmonary artery and the aortic valve between the left ventricle and aorta. Semilunar valves viewed from above appear like three crescent moons.

71. D: Improper electrode placement is the most common cause of excessive artifacts in EKG tracings. Improper placement can include loose electrodes, dried conductive gel, inadequate skin preparation, and lead mispositioning. Studies have shown that mispositioning occurs in up to 4% of EKGs. Mispositioning of the precordial leads can lead to misinterpretation as a myocardial infarct. It is important to determine if the EKG machine uses the US or the European color-coding system and to follow best practices in applying the electrodes.

72. C: All of the listed irregularities are types of arrhythmias. This pattern is seen in ventricular tachycardia, which is a very fast heart rate originating in the ventricles. Both ventricular tachycardia and ventricular fibrillation, which looks like an irregular up-and-down pattern on an EKG, can indicate myocardial infarction and life-threatening situations. Atrial fibrillation can be associated with conditions like mitral valve prolapse, and is indicated on an EKG by irregularly spaced patterns without distinguishable P waves. Paroxysmal atrial tachycardia is a sudden pattern of more rapid beating that lasts briefly; it can be seen in cardiac patients but often occurs in healthy people.

73. D: This EKG tracing indicates ventricular fibrillation, a life-threatening arrhythmia. If the patient was awake and responsive when this rhythm presented, then the technician could check the patient's pulse and check the electrodes and leads first, but since the patient lost consciousness and is unresponsive, the first action should be to call for help following facility protocol and begin basic life support until relieved by other healthcare providers. Because ventricular fibrillation is a shockable rhythm, the EKG technician should expect that the patient will require defibrillation.

74. C: Isopropyl alcohol 70% wipes are appropriate to use to disinfect lead wires and EKG machine surfaces. Sodium hypochlorite >10% (undiluted bleach) may cause corrosion to the insulation on lead wires. If bleach is used, then it must be diluted to a 1:10 solution and must be wiped off thoroughly. Hydrogen peroxide in concentrations greater than 3% may degrade plastic and rubber materials. Ammonia-based cleaners should be avoided since they can damage the EKG screen coating and the lead wire insulation.

75. A: Leads I, II, and III are bipolar leads because they detect the voltage difference in electrical potential between two electrodes, with one electrode being positive and the other negative. Leads aVR, aVL, aVF, V1, V2, V3, V4, V5, and V6 are unipolar leads. These leads measure electrical potential at one positive electrode relative to a central point of reference. Both types of leads provide information about the heart that is essential for diagnosis and accurate cardiac assessment.

76. C, D, E: Patch monitors are typically left in place for 7–14 days, so patients are allowed to shower and bathe after 24 hours but should avoid direct water on the device. The patients should also avoid activities that cause excess sweating, which may loosen the device, and they should avoid placing an electric blanket over the patch for the same reason. Patients should be advised to press the button on the device to indicate adverse events and to report any itching or skin irritation.

77. D: For adults and children 1 year and older the best place to check for a pulse with suspected cardiac arrest is the carotid artery since it has the strongest pulse because it is close to the heart, it is easy to locate because it is a large artery, and it is less affected by the peripheral vasoconstriction that often occurs. For infants younger than 1 year old, the brachial pulse is the easiest to locate because the infant's neck is short and often chubby, and pressing to try to locate the carotid pulse may compress the infant's airway.

78. C: Einthoven's triangle is a theoretical inverted equidistant triangle that represents the electrical activity of the heart formed by three standard limb leads (i.e., leads I, II, and III) and the RA, LA, and LL electrodes. The heart lies at the center, and the RL electrode does not contribute because it is the neutral (or ground) electrode. According to Einthoven's law, the electrical potential of leads I and II is equal to that of lead III.

79. C: A Holter monitor is worn for 24–48 hours to help evaluate for the presence of arrhythmias. In the event that a significant arrhythmia is detected, a pacemaker may need to be placed. It cannot evaluate the structures of the heart.

80. C: The medical term for a heart attack is a myocardial infarction. A heart attack occurs when the cardiac cells in a portion of the heart die due to prolonged insufficient blood and oxygen flow. Signs and symptoms may include chest pain, shortness of breath, palpitations, diaphoresis, nausea, vomiting, dizziness, and feeling of impending doom.

81. D: If a patient has or may have a highly transmissible disease, both Standard Precautions and the applicable type of Transmission-Based Precautions should be used. Transmission-Based Precautions depend on whether the infectious disease is spread via the airborne route, physical contact, or respiratory droplets. The hallmark of Standard Precautions is use of personal protective equipment, which includes gloves, gowns, and mouth, nose, and eye protection, but they also include proper hand hygiene, as well as care with other potentially infectious materials, such as laundry.

82. A: Occupational Safety and Health Administration (OSHA) was signed into law by President Richard Nixon in 1970. It was established to ensure that employees are provided with the training necessary to perform their job duties safely while offering a safe work environment in which to do so. The agency is also responsible for protection to employees who enact the whistleblower action to report unsafe conditions at the place of their employment.

83. D: Wellens' syndrome is characterized by T waves that are deeply inverted or biphasic following an episode of chest pain. During the episode of acute pain, the abnormal T waves are often not observed, so patients with a history of recent chest pain should have a follow-up EKG when the pain subsides. Wellens' syndrome is an indication of stenosis of the left anterior descending artery. Wellens' syndrome is sometimes referred to as the "widow-maker" sign because it often progresses to a major ST-segment elevation myocardial infarction within a short period.

84. A: If a patient has a Holter monitor (lead type), the patient should avoid showering, bathing, or swimming for the duration of use (typically 24–48 hours) because the electrodes must be kept dry, or they may loosen and dislodge, resulting in a loss of signal or artifacts. Additionally, most lead-type Holter monitors are not designed to be waterproof. Patch-type monitors, such as the Zio patch, however, can typically be worn in the shower after 24 hours, although water sprayed directly against the device should be avoided. The Zio patch adheres with a hydrocolloid adhesive.

85. B: The preferred disposal method is to put the sharp directly into a sharps container after use. Sharps and other biohazard containers have an orange or red-orange biohazard sticker. The scoop technique is a way to recap the needle for transport only if the sharps container is not nearby. Sharps and other forms of infectious waste are later burned or sterilized before disposal, usually by a company specializing in this disposal.

86. A: In an EKG tracing, the QRS complex represents ventricular depolarization, which is the wave of conduction moving across the ventricles. The P-wave indicates the depolarization wave initiated by the SA node and is followed by the QRS complex, with the Q wave showing a downward deflection and the R wave showing an upward deflection. The T wave, which immediately follows the QRS complex, represents repolarization, reverting to a state of readiness for the next wave of conduction.

87. C:

Electrode	US (AHA)	Europe (IEC)
RA	White	Red
LA	Black	Yellow
RL	Green	Black
LL	Red	Green
V1	Red	Red
V2	Yellow	Yellow
V3	Green	Green
V4	Blue	Brown
V5	Orange	Black
V6	Purple	Violet

88. C: With three-lead EKG monitoring, the right arm (white) and left arm (black) electrodes are typically placed on the corresponding side on the upper torso, below the clavicle at the midclavicular line. The left leg (red) electrode is place on the left lower torso. This placement allows the patient to move more easily and also provides a more accurate EKG tracing. This configuration forms three bipolar leads: lead I, lead II, and lead III. The three-lead configuration is used for cardiac telemetry, basic heart assessment during transport, monitoring during anesthesia, and Holter monitoring.

89. A: The normal oxygen saturation at rest is 95–100%; a drop of the oxygen saturation level of 4% or more from baseline during exercise is significant. If the patient's oxygen saturation level is 86% at rest, then the healthcare provider should be consulted before proceeding. In some cases, patients whose oxygen saturation levels are lower than normal or whose levels fall sharply during exercise may undergo testing while receiving oxygen. This may be done to help determine the patient's need for supplementary oxygen during activities.

90. A: The Karvonen/Heart rate reserve (HRR) method to determine the target heart rate (THR) involves first determining the maximum heart rate (MHR) and the resting heart rate (RHR) (the first noted in the morning). Below is the formula for a 70-year-old patient with an RHR of 82 and exercise intensity of 50%:

- MHR – RHR = HRR
- HRR × exercise intensity percentage
- Add the RHR

Using the Fox & Haskell method for MHR:

- 220 – 70 (age) = 150 MHR – 82 (RHR) = 68 (HRR)
- 68 × 0.50 (exercise intensity) = 34
- 34 + 82 = 116 THR

91. B: The intrinsic rate of the SA node is between 60 and 100 bpm, and it serves as the primary pacemaker of the heart. If the SA node fails, the AV node serves as a backup, but its intrinsic rate is lower, at 40–60 bpm. This rate can still generally provide adequate circulation. However, if the AV node fails, then the Purkinje fibers or ventricular myocytes in the ventricles are forced to take over, but their intrinsic rate is only 20–40 bpm—this rate cannot effectively sustain life.

92. C: Line number two is the thorax sternal line. The midsternal line runs down the middle of the sternum, while the sternal line runs along the lateral border of the sternum. The V1 and V2 electrodes are placed along the parasternal line, which runs parallel to the sternal line. The midclavicular line runs down the chest from the midpoint of the clavicle, while the anterior axillary line runs vertically along the anterior axillary fold.

93. C: Orthopnea is a condition in which the patient becomes short of breath when lying flat. These patients are typically placed in semi-Fowler's position (30–45 degrees) for the EKG. Fowler's positions include:

- Low semi-Fowler's: 15–30 degrees, used during postsurgical recovery
- Semi-Fowler's: 30–45 degrees, used for support of respirations and to reduce aspiration risk
- Standard Fowler's: 45–60 degrees, used for increased respiratory distress, heart failure
- High/Full Fowler's: 60–90 degrees, used for severe respiratory distress, heart failure.

94. A: If a patient's skin is very hairy, this can prevent the electrodes from adhering properly and can lead to artifacts or poor signal. The best method of removing hair is by using clippers because they can cut the hair close to the skin. Shaving may cause small cuts in the skin, which increase the risk of infection and irritation, and depilatories may be irritating to the skin. The hair should be clipped only in areas of individual electrode placement.

95. B: A 15-lead EKG for a pediatric patient requires 3 additional electrodes:

- V3R: Midway between V1 and V4R on the right chest
- V4R: Below the nipple line, at the midclavicular line on the right chest
- V7: On the left postaxillary line level with V6
- Limb electrodes should not be placed on the torso. The RA and LA electrodes should be placed just above the elbows and the RL and LA electrodes between the ankle and the knee.

96. A: With atrial flutter, as in the EKG tracing, the sawtooth waves that occur are referred to as flutter (F) waves, indicating rapid atrial depolarizations. Flutter waves can affect the appearance of the T wave. In some cases, the T waves are completely obscured by the F waves, especially if the heart rate is rapid. The T waves may be present but distorted and may merge with the F waves, resulting in a sawtooth appearance.

97. A: The sequence recommended by the CDC for PPE removal is gown and gloves (together), then goggles, then mask, and finally washing the hands. This process is optimal for ensuring the prevention of exposure to pathogens. If taking off gown and gloves separately, gloves should be removed before the gown. After each type of PPE is removed, it should be disposed of in a biohazard container.

98. A, B, E: Pulse oximeters are usually placed on an index finger to monitor oxygen saturation, but a number of different factors can interfere with accurate readings:

- Impaired circulation can decrease blood flow to the hands.
- If the hands are very cold, the blood vessels may constrict.
- Dark nail polish can interfere with accuracy because the pulse oximeter uses light absorption to measure oxygen saturation.
- Fluorescent lights or other bright lights may alter readings.
- Tremors or excessive movement may disrupt measurement of light absorption.

Answer Key and Explanations for Test #2

99. B: Blood flows into the heart from the superior and inferior vena cava into the right atrium and through the tricuspid valve to the right ventricle. From there, the blood goes through the pulmonic valve into the pulmonary artery and to the lungs for oxygenation. Oxygenated blood returns through the pulmonary artery to the left atrium and then through the mitral valve to the left ventricle. The left ventricle then pumps the blood through the aortic valve into the aorta and general circulation.

100. D: All adult patients should be treated as though they are adults; however, patients with developmental disabilities, such as trisomy 21 (Down syndrome) or with dementia (such as Alzheimer's disease) often benefit from having a parent or caregiver accompany them into the testing area and stay with them during testing. This is especially true if patients are obviously upset or frightened because they may be uncooperative and resistive during the EKG exam. The EKG technician should give the patient time to calm down and should reassure the patient that the EKG does not hurt.

EKG Tech Practice Test #3

1. If using the FAST mnemonic to remember the signs of a stroke, what does the F stand for?

    a. Face drooping
    b. Failure to respond
    c. Favoring one side
    d. Fine tremors

2. The electrode placement shown in the diagram below is commonly used for:

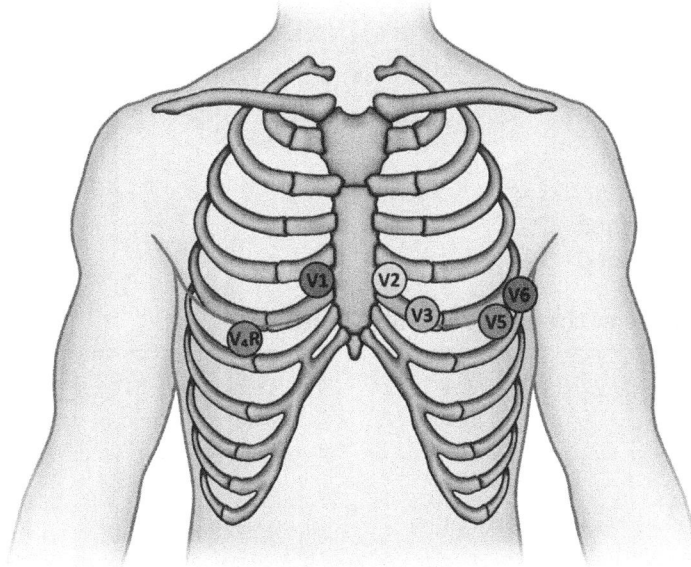

    a. Neonates
    b. Children younger than age 5
    c. Adolescents
    d. Frail older adults

3. Describe the duration, amplitude, and appearance of the P waves in the following EKG tracing:

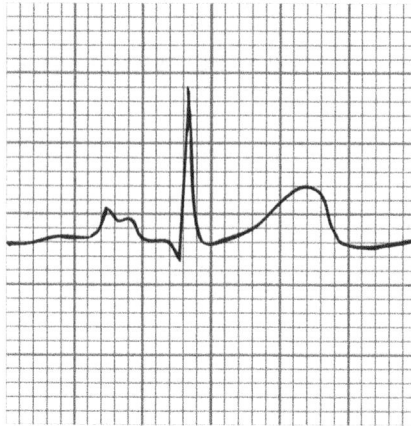

a. 0.28 sec, 3 mm, rounded
b. 0.09 sec, 2 mm, peaked
c. 0.12 sec, 1 mm, notched
d. 0.12 sec, 2 mm, notched

4. What is likely the cause of the following EKG finding?

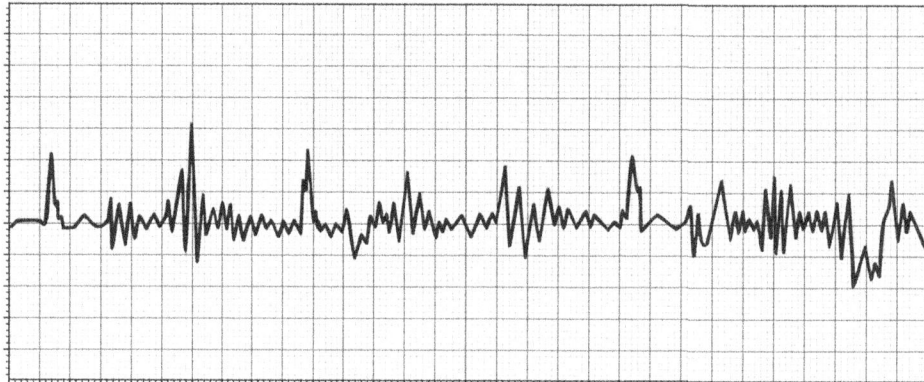

a. Electrical interference artifact
b. Dislodged electrode
c. Somatic tremor artifact
d. Broken recording

5. What is the average body temperature in a human (in Fahrenheit)?

a. 96.8 degrees.
b. 100 degrees.
c. 98.6 degrees.
d. 37 degrees.

6. When taking the pulse rate for children up to 5 years old, which of the following is the preferred pulse site?

    a. Radial pulse
    b. Brachial pulse
    c. Apical pulse
    d. Dorsalis pedis pulse

7. hat is the approximate heart rate in the following EKG tracing?

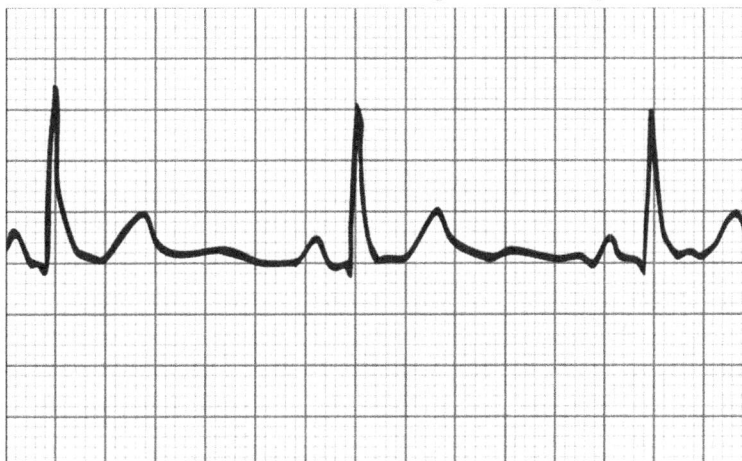

    a. 60
    b. 55
    c. 50
    d. 45

8. What do the P waves on the following EKG strip indicate?

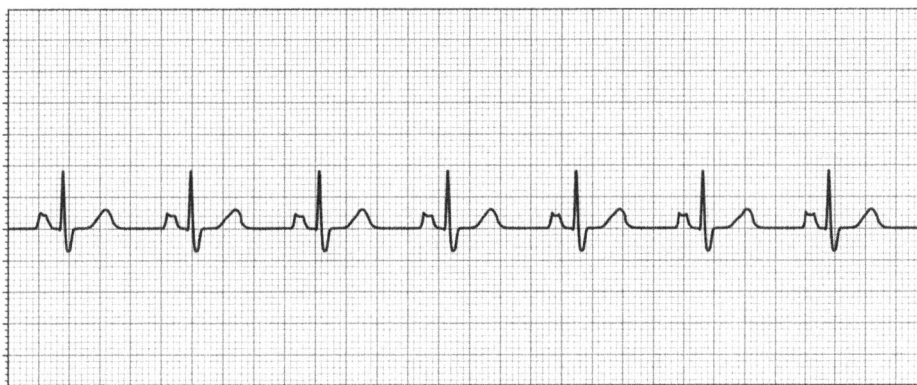

    a. Normal variation
    b. Left atrial enlargement
    c. Right atrial enlargement
    d. Right ventricular enlargement

EKG Tech Practice Test #3

9. If a patient is lying on their back, they are in a _____ position.

    a. Prone
    b. Prostrate
    c. Dorsal
    d. Supine

10. Which of the following circumstances may warrant changing the speed of the EKG to 50 mm/sec? (Select the three [3] correct answers.)

    a. Infants' and young children's EKGs
    b. Older adults' EKGs
    c. Supraventricular tachycardia (SVT)
    d. Atrial flutter
    e. Bradycardia

11. Which of the following is FALSE regarding Occupational Safety and Health Administration (OSHA)?

    a. Employers must inform workers of work hazards through training.
    b. Employers must protect employees from discrimination if they report work hazards.
    c. Employers must provide employees with free personal protective gear.
    d. Employers must provide employees with job benefits and vacation time.

12. Which of the following cannot be detected by a 12-lead EKG?

    a. Rhythm.
    b. Ischemia.
    c. Vegetation.
    d. Rate.

13. A coworker has been spotted throwing someone's medical record in the trash can in the break room. Which of the following is not an appropriate course of action?

    a. Report the action to your supervisor.
    b. Ignore the coworker's actions.
    c. Confront the coworker.
    d. Remove the records from the trash.

14. A patient has a small (4.5 cm length) implanted cardiac monitor in the chest at the normal site for the V2 electrode placement. The EKG technician should:

    a. Place the electrode above the implant.
    b. Place the electrode in its usual position.
    c. Place the electrode to the left side of the implant.
    d. Place the electrode to the right of the V3 electrode.

15. What type of heart block does this EKG tracing demonstrate?

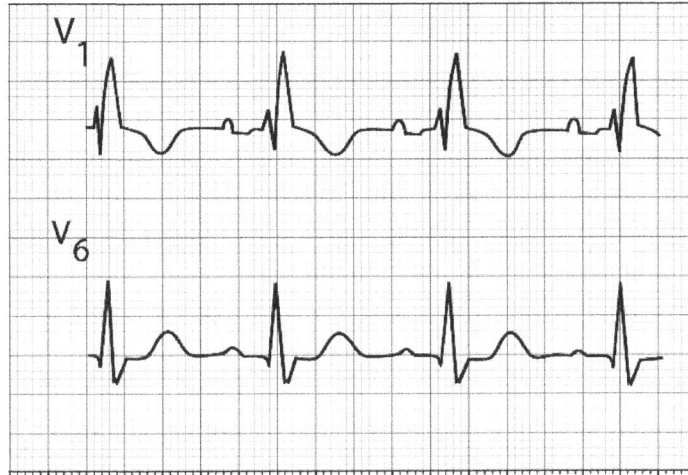

a. First-degree AV block
b. Second-degree AV block (Mobitz I)
c. Right bundle branch block
d. Left bundle branch block

16. When taking a standard EKG, where should the bipolar leads be placed?

a. Between the left and right arms, the left leg and right arm, and the left leg and left arm
b. Between the middle of the left arm to left leg and the right arm, the middle of the right arm to left leg and the left arm, and the middle of the right arm to left arm and the left leg
c. Between six different points on the chest and a point on the right arm to left leg lead
d. Between six different points on the chest and the intersection of the left arm/right arm/left leg leads

17. The EKG technician is capturing an EKG and, upon review, notes an abnormal rhythm. The rhythm starts with a normal looking P wave followed by a normal QRS complex, but the distance between the P wave and QRS complex gets progressively longer with each beat. There also appears to be a missing QRS complex before a seemingly normal P wave and QRS complex return. What rhythm is the EKG technician seeing?

a. First-degree heart block
b. Second-degree type I (Mobitz type I) heart block
c. Second-degree type II (Mobitz type II) heart block
d. Third-degree heart block

18. If a patient who is to wear a Holter monitor for 24 hours also has an implanted pacemaker, what is generally the minimum safe distance between the pacemaker and the recorder?

a. 12 inches
b. 10 inches
c. 8 inches
d. 6 inches

19. The Lewis lead EKG modification is typically done to:
a. Detect right ventricular infarcts
b. Adjust for obesity
c. Enhance detection of atrial activity
d. Identify posterior wall infarcts

20. When interviewing a patient, which of the following types of question prompts only a yes or no response?
a. Indirect statement
b. Closed question
c. Open-ended question
d. Active question

21. Which type of electrode placement is used for a 12-month-old infant?
a. Right-sided
b. Standard left-sided
c. Posterior
d. Lower limb

22. If a patient with an implanted cardiac monitor goes into cardiac arrest, the defibrillator paddles should not be placed closer than:
a. 3 inches from the battery pack
b. 5 inches from the battery pack
c. 6 inches from the battery pack
d. 7 inches from the battery pack

23. What is the MOST common blood-borne illness in the United States?
a. Roseola.
b. AIDS.
c. Varicella.
d. Hepatitis C.

24. Which of the following best describes universal precautions?
a. Treating human body fluids as if they contained infectious diseases.
b. Medical precautions taken when traveling abroad.
c. Ensuring the vaccination of all children.
d. The use of prophylactic medications.

25. If an EKG tracing is taken at the default speed with standard gain, the calibration mark should be:
a. 10 mm (1 mV) high and 5 mm (0.2 sec) wide
b. 5 mm (0.5 mV) high and 5 mm (0.2 sec) wide
c. 10 mm (1 mV) high and 10 mm (0.4 sec) wide
d. 5 mm (0.5 mV) high and 10 mm (0.4 sec) wide

26. **Which of the following adequately describes the qualities necessary for active listening?**
    a. Being alert and interested in what the other person is saying
    b. Maintaining eye contact with the other person
    c. Being attuned to what is said and what is communicated nonverbally
    d. Being able to respond quickly with a corrective action

27. **The precordial leads in a 12-lead EKG record electrical activity in the:**
    a. Frontal plane
    b. Sagittal plane
    c. Median plane
    d. Horizontal plane

28. **Which of the following is an example of objective data when documenting?**
    a. Patient is unable to recall his or her birthdate or home address.
    b. Patient is upset about the wait time.
    c. Patient feels well.
    d. Patient is depressed.

29. **The EKG changes that are common to myocardial injury and myocardial infarction include:**
    a. ST segment elevation and T-wave inversion
    b. ST segment depression and T-wave inversion
    c. Prolonged QT segment with T-wave inversion
    d. T-wave inversion and absent P wave

30. **What is the most accurate measurement of body temperature?**
    a. Rectal.
    b. Axillary.
    c. Temporal.
    d. Oral.

31. **Which of the following health care issues is NOT covered under the Health Insurance Portability and Accountability Act (HIPAA)?**
    a. Increasing the portability of health insurance
    b. Addressing health care fraud and abuse
    c. Standardizing the electronic transmission of health data
    d. Outlining payment of Medicare and Medicaid

32. **If a patient has an implanted pacemaker for ventricular pacing, the EKG technician should expect that the pacing spike on the EKG strip will:**
    a. Precede the P wave
    b. Precede the QRS complex
    c. Precede the T wave
    d. Appear at random

33. When monitoring a patient during an exercise stress test, the EKG technician would expect that for every increase in the level of exertion, the patient's heart rate will increase by:

    a. 5 bpm
    b. 10 bpm
    c. 15 bpm
    d. 20 bpm

34. What is another term for advance directive?

    a. Living will.
    b. Power of attorney.
    c. Estate representative.
    d. Legal guardian.

35. A primary difference between pulsed VT and pulseless ventricular tachycardia is that with pulseless VT:

    a. The patient is unresponsive.
    b. The P wave is absent.
    c. The QRS complex is narrow.
    d. The rate is more irregular.

36. The type of pacemaker malfunction that the following EKG demonstrates is:

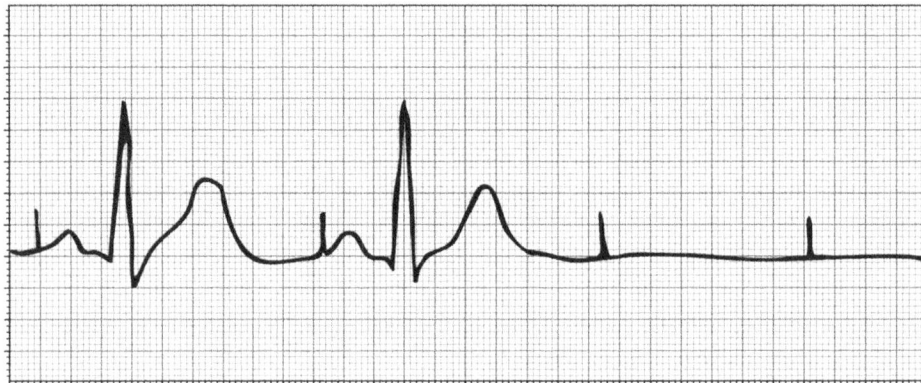

    a. No malfunction
    b. Failure to sense
    c. Failure to capture
    d. Failure to pace

37. If an EKG order calls for Mason-Likar EKG electrode placement, this involves:

    a. Changing the position of all leads
    b. Placing the limb lead on the upper chest and lower torso
    c. Changing the position of the precordial leads
    d. Placing the limb leads on the upper arm and thigh

38. What is the rhythm in the following EKG strip?

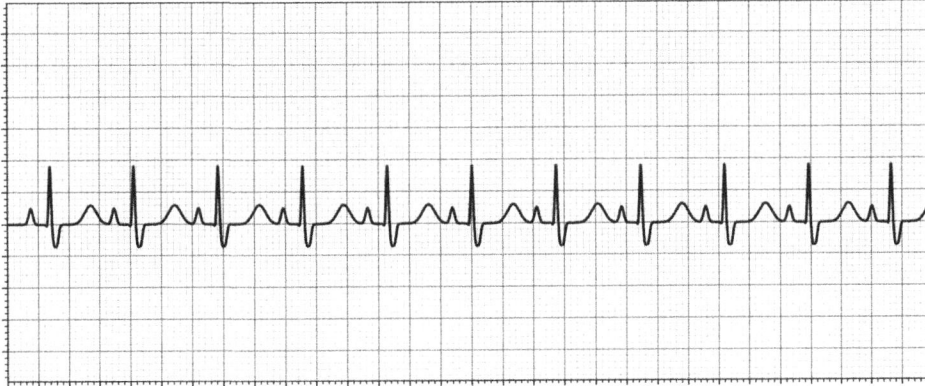

a. Sinus tachycardia
b. Normal sinus rhythm
c. Atrial tachycardia
d. Junctional escape rhythm

39. The following EKG tracing is an example of which one of the following?

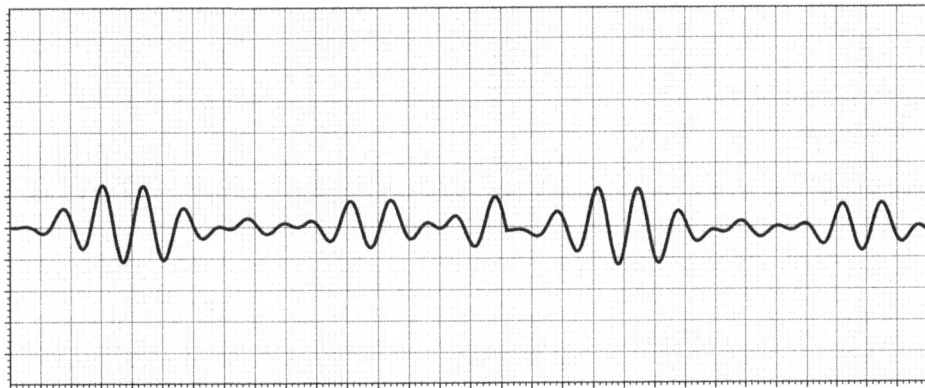

a. Ventricular fibrillation
b. Torsades de pointes
c. VT
d. Accelerated idioventricular rhythm

40. What type of sinoatrial (SA) block does the following EKG tracing demonstrate?

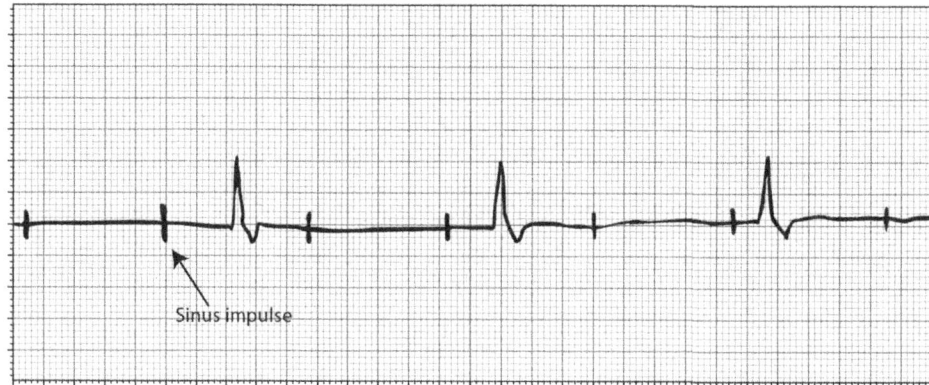

Sinus impulse

a. First-degree SA block
b. Second-degree SA block, type I
c. Second-degree SA block, type II
d. Third-degree SA block

41. What piece of equipment measures oxygen saturation?

a. Foley catheter.
b. Urometer.
c. Sphygmomanometer.
d. Pulse oximeter.

42. With reversal of electrodes V1 and V2, the EKG technician should notice that:

a. V1 has a smaller R wave than V2.
b. V1 and V2 have the same size R waves.
c. The R waves are missing in V1.
d. V1 has a larger R wave than V2.

43. When positioning a Zio XT patch monitor, the arrow on the top label should point:

a. To the right
b. To the left
c. Up
d. Down

44. An EKG shows the occasional P wave that is not followed by a QRS complex. When the P wave is followed by a QRS complex, the P-R interval is consistent. What does the EKG demonstrate?

a. First-degree AV block
b. Second-degree heart block (Mobitz type I)
c. Second-degree heart block (Mobitz type II)
d. Sinus pause

45. What is the Q-T interval on the following EKG tracing?

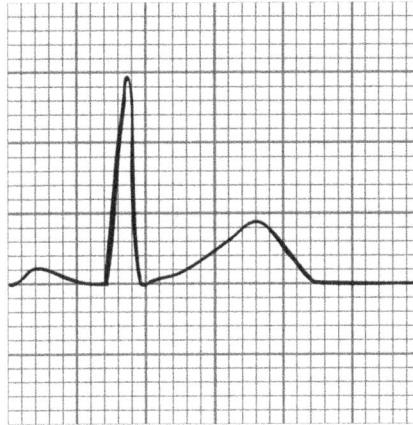

    a. 0.28 mm
    b. 0.42 mm
    c. 0.60 mm
    d. 0.68 mm

46. A patient with a probable cardiovascular or respiratory problem should be positioned on the examination table in what position?

    a. Dorsal recumbent or lithotomy
    b. Semi- or high Fowler's
    c. Trendelenburg
    d. Sims'

47. Which of the following is an external barrier to communication?

    a. Weather.
    b. Pain.
    c. Hunger.
    d. Anger.

48. Which represents a normal heart rate in an adult human?

    a. 20 beats per minute.
    b. 60 beats per minute.
    c. 120 beats per minute.
    d. 160 beats per minute.

49. A late-term pregnant woman is scheduled for a 12-lead EKG. In what position should the patient be placed?

    a. Supine
    b. Left lateral tilt
    c. High semi-Fowler's
    d. Reverse Trendelenburg

50. What is the medical term for a respiratory rate of 32 breaths per minute?

  a. Bradycardia.
  b. Tachypnea.
  c. Tachycardia.
  d. Bradypnea.

51. Which of the following best describes the current American Heart Association guidelines for emergency cardiopulmonary resuscitation (CPR) on an adult?

  a. Perform rescue breathing using one breath every 10 seconds.
  b. For circulation, use a ratio of 30 fast compressions to two breaths.
  c. Shock with an automated external defibrillator (AED) prior to CPR.
  d. Initiate CPR starting with rescue breaths followed by compressions.

52. What are standard precautions?

  a. Guidelines about protecting yourself from a potentially aggressive patient
  b. Guidelines about how to set up an office for patient and employee safety
  c. Guidelines about how to prevent patients from suing
  d. Guidelines about protecting yourself from potential infection

53. What electrodes are typically applied for a transthoracic echocardiogram?

  a. V1, V2, and V3
  b. RA, LA, and V1
  c. RA, LA, and LL
  d. V1, V2, and RA

54. If there are 25 small boxes (5 large boxes) between R waves, what is the heart rate using the sequencing method?

  a. 100
  b. 75
  c. 60
  d. 50

55. Which of the following reflects a normal QRS complex?

  a. 0.08 seconds.
  b. 0.80 seconds.
  c. 2.0 seconds.
  d. 0.20 seconds.

56. According to the OSHA Bloodborne Pathogens Standard, what is required if an employee is accidentally exposed to blood or other potentially infectious materials?

  a. The employer must conduct an immediate medical evaluation of the employee.
  b. The incident must be reported to a superior and documented within 48 hours.
  c. The employer must offer to test the employee for HBV, HCV, and HIV.
  d. The employer must submit an ISO 9001 form.

57. What is the duration of the Q-T interval in the following tracing?

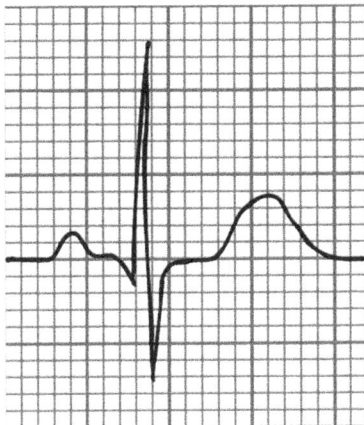

a. 0.60 sec
b. 0.48 sec
c. 0.52 sec
d. 0.40 sec

58. A patient with a blood pressure of 165/81 mm Hg has what condition?

a. Tachycardia.
b. Hypotension.
c. Hypertension.
d. Tachypnea.

59. Which one of the following choices is a shockable rhythm?

a. Asystole
b. Atrial fibrillation
c. Pulseless ventricular tachycardia (VT)
d. Pulseless electrical activity

60. On the EKG tracing, the T wave represents:

a. Atrial depolarization
b. Ventricular depolarization
c. Atrial repolarization
d. Ventricular repolarization

61. What does the P wave represent?

a. Atrial repolarization
b. Atrial depolarization
c. Ventricular repolarization
d. Ventricular depolarization

62. If a patient suffers a cardiac arrest during an EKG, and a healthcare professional has brought the automated external defibrillator (AED), the EKG technician should:

a. Assist in applying the AED defibrillator pads.
b. Remove the EKG electrodes.
c. Stand aside.
d. Ask what to do.

63. What type of pacemaker malfunction is demonstrated by the following EKG tracing?

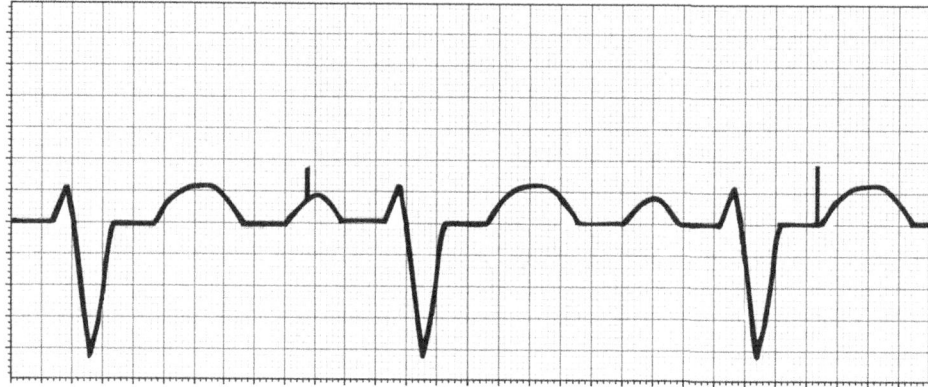

a. No malfunction
b. Failure to sense
c. Failure to capture
d. Failure to pace

64.

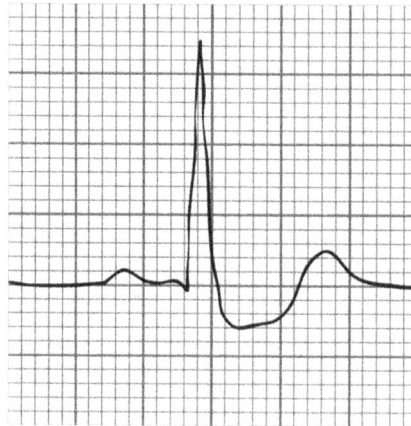

What is notable about the EKG tracing above?

a. Prolonged P wave
b. Narrow QRS complex
c. ST segment elevation
d. ST segment depression

65. Touching a patient in a manner to which they have not consented is considered a tort of:

a. Invasion of privacy
b. Battery
c. Libel
d. Slander

66. A patient's chart indicates dextrocardia, a right-sided heart. To perform an EKG exam, the correct electrode placement for V1 is at the:

    a.   Fourth intercostal space, right of the sternum
    b.   Fourth intercostal space, left of the sternum
    c.   Third intercostal space, right of the sternum
    d.   Fifth intercostal space, left of the sternum

67. If a patient is to have an EKG exam in a hospital bed, once the electrodes are applied, how should the siderails be positioned?

    a.   Upper and bottom siderails raised
    b.   Upper siderails raised, lower siderails down
    c.   Upper siderail lowered on side of the EKG technician, lower siderails down
    d.   Upper siderail lowered on side of the EKG technician, lower siderails raised

68. A patient has had a left total mastectomy, and the scar extends over the usual V2 to V6 electrode positions. Where should the EKG technician place the electrodes for an EKG?

    a.   On the scar in the usual positions
    b.   On the right side of the chest in mirrored positions
    c.   Above the scar in approximate positions
    d.   Below the scar in approximate positions

69. If the hospital uses a radiofrequency system for wireless telemetry, the patient should typically be advised to stay within what range of the monitor to ensure that the signal is detected?

    a.   30–100 feet
    b.   300–1,000 feet
    c.   1,000 2,000 feet
    d.   Unlimited throughout the facility regardless of its size

70. Which of the following are potentially lethal dysrhythmias? (Select the three [3] correct answers.)

    a.   First-degree AV block
    b.   VT
    c.   Agonal rhythm
    d.   Sinus arrhythmia
    e.   Ventricular fibrillation

71. HIPAA (Health Insurance Portability and Accountability Act) regulations apply to which of the following?

    a.   Physicians.
    b.   Secretaries.
    c.   Clinical documentation specialists.
    d.   All employees of a healthcare facility.

72. Which of the following would NOT facilitate communication with a geriatric patient?

    a.   Using clear terminology.
    b.   Repeating important phrases.
    c.   Speaking slowly.
    d.   Keeping the voice low.

73. Which represents a normal pulse oximetry reading on room air?

    a. 100 percent.
    b. 90 percent.
    c. 75 percent.
    d. 50 percent.

74. The most effective method of checking whether the rhythm on an EKG tracing is regular or irregular is to:

    a. Count the small boxes.
    b. Use a ruler to measure.
    c. Use a marked piece of paper.
    d. Use calipers.

75. For the five-lead EKG, where are the RL and LL electrodes placed?

    a. On the right and left lower legs
    b. On the right and left upper legs
    c. On the right and left lower chest
    d. On the right and left lower abdomen

76. Which of the following telemetry alarms are generally considered high priority?

    a. Atrial fibrillation (new onset)
    b. Infrequent premature ventricular contractions (PVCs)
    c. Tachycardia (short run)
    d. Severe bradycardia

77. Which of the following is not part of nonverbal communication?

    a. Facial expression.
    b. Eye contact.
    c. Tone of voice.
    d. Posture.

78. The OSHA Bloodborne Pathogens Standard applies to contact with:

    a. Blood and all body fluids
    b. Blood and all body fluids, secretions, and excretions
    c. The items in response B plus non-intact skin and mucous membranes
    d. The items in response C plus unfixed human tissue and tissue culture, cells, or fluid known to be positive for HIV, HBV, or HCV

79. A patient who is chronically homeless may have difficulties effectively communicating because of which of the following internal barriers?

    a. Anger.
    b. Pain.
    c. Hunger.
    d. Sadness.

80. What information is not included in the history of present illness section of a medical chart?

a. Onset of symptoms.
b. Pain scale.
c. Associated symptoms.
d. Physical exam.

81. If using the five heart rates zones to determine the intensity level for exercise, at which zone should the patient be comfortable and able to talk easily?

a. Zone 1
b. Zone 2
c. Zone 3
d. Zone 4

82. If a patient passes out during an exercise test and the EKG technician is able to find a pulse and observe normal respirations but the patient remains unconscious, in what position should the patient be placed?

a. Trendelenburg
b. Supine
c. Prone
d. Lateral recumbent

83. Which type of escape rhythm is characterized by absent or inverted P waves, short P-R interval, narrow QRS complex, and a heart rate of 40–60 bpm?

a. Ventricular
b. Junctional
c. Accelerated junctional
d. Accelerated idioventricular

84. What EKG setup is typically used for basic EKG monitoring for patients in emergency transport?

a. 3-lead
b. 5-lead
c. 7-lead
d. 12-lead

85. Before attaching the lead wires to a Holter monitor, the EKG technician should:

a. Connect the electrodes to the lead wires.
b. Check the batteries.
c. Apply the electrodes.
d. Fasten the belt clip.

86. Which of the following best describes ethics?

a. Individual choices relating to conduct
b. Personal values governing an individual's perceptions of right and wrong
c. Laws defining acceptable behavior
d. Creeds to live by

EKG Tech Practice Test #3

87. How should a blood pressure measurement be recorded on an adult patient's chart?

a. Systolic pressure/diastolic pressure
b. Systolic pressure/diastolic pressure, arm used, patient position
c. Diastolic pressure/systolic pressure
d. Diastolic pressure/systolic pressure, arm used, patient position

88. What distinguishes polymorphic VT from monomorphic VT?

a. The QRS complexes vary in shape and amplitude
b. The heart rate ranges from 150 to 250 bpm
c. The p wave may be absent or not associated with the QRS complex
d. The P-R interval is absent

89. What abnormality is evident on the following EKG tracing?

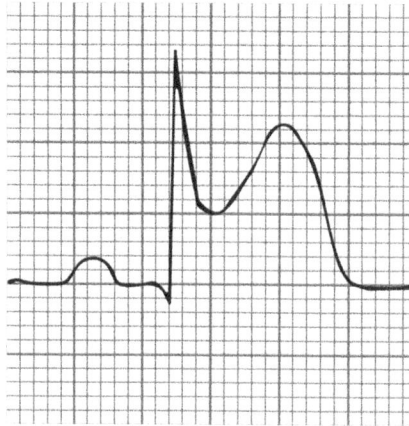

a. Tented T waves
b. QRS slurring
c. U waves
d. Elevated ST segment

90. The combination of various sources into a comprehensive electronic database for patient information is known as a(n):

a. Electronic medical record (EMR)
b. Electronic health record (EHR)
c. Medical office simulation software (MOSS)
d. Total practice management system (TPMS)

91. If a patient is to have a seven-lead configuration for ambulatory monitoring with a Holter monitor, what additional electrodes are used?

a. V2 and V3
b. V3 and V4
c. V2 and V5
d. V3 and V5

92. All of the following abnormalities of respiration are associated with a period of complete absence of breathing EXCEPT:

a. Voluntarily holding one's breath
b. Orthopnea
c. Sleep apnea
d. Cheyne-Stokes respiration

93. An EKG strip mounting sheet has three horizontal columns with room for four strips.

Lead I	Lead II	Lead III

On the first vertical column, which begins with lead I, which leads should follow vertically?

a. aVR, V1, and V4
b. aVL V2, and V6
c. aVF, V1, and V2
d. aVF, V3, and V6

94. If an EKG machine uses Z-fold thermal paper, when loading a new supply, it is important to first:

a. Fan the Z-fold stack.
b. Remove any jammed or leftover sheets.
c. Ensure that the printed side faces down.
d. Trim the paper edges.

95. During an exercise stress test, a patient complains of feeling severe "pressure" in the chest; the EKG technician should recognize this as a possible sign of:

a. Heart attack
b. Hypertension
c. Anxiety
d. Reflux

96. Which of the following nonverbal cues display empathy?

a. Relaxed posture, loud voice, limited eye contact.
b. Rigid posture, low voice, limited eye contact.
c. Relaxed posture, low voice, consistent eye contact.
d. Rigid posture, loud voice, consistent eye contact.

97. The P waves on the following EKG tracing (lead II) are an indication of:

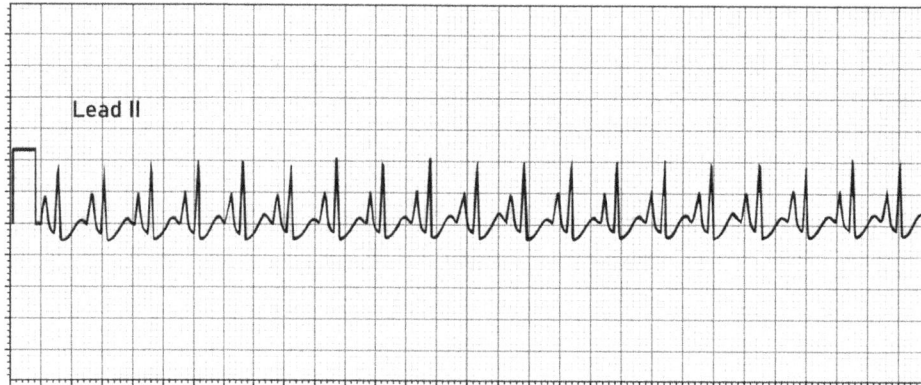

a. Left atrial enlargement
b. Right atrial enlargement
c. Ectopic atrial rhythm
d. Multifocal atrial tachycardia

98. When interpreting an EKG, the first step is generally to:
a. Analyze the rhythm.
b. Determine the heart rate.
c. Note the presence or absence of a P wave.
d. Assess the QRS complex.

99. What should you do if you become aware that a colleague is working while intoxicated?
a. Approach the colleague and warn them not to do it again.
b. Report the situation to your supervisor.
c. Make sure the colleague enters an appropriate treatment program.
d. Tell your other coworkers so you can work as a group to ensure that the colleague is able to perform his or her job sufficiently.

100. The major difference between electronic and other types of sphygmomanometers used to measure blood pressure is that electronic types:
a. Do not use a pressure cuff
b. Do not require simultaneous use of a stethoscope
c. Tend to lose calibration and accuracy
d. Can only read systole or diastole measurements in one take

Answer Key and Explanations for Test #3

1. A: The FAST mnemonic to remember the signs of a stroke:

F	Face drooping	One side of the face droops; a lopsided smile.
A	Arm weak	One side of the body may be weak, paralyzed, or numb. If the patient is standing, the patient may fall or have difficulty trying to walk.
S	Speech difficulty	Speech may be slurred, confused, or may be unable to speak or understand speech. The patient may be unable to follow directions.
T	Time to call for help	Immediate treatment, within 60 minutes if possible, is essential to prevent long-term disability. Patients should be transported to an emergency department if outside of the hospital.

2. B: The electrode placement that moves V4 from the left to the right is typically used for children younger than age 5 (most often ages 2–5 or older depending on size). V4R is placed in a mirrored position to where V4 would normally be placed on the left side, at the fifth intercostal space on the right midclavicular line. This placement is used because the right ventricle has not yet moved from the right side of the sternum. This V4R lead must be clearly labeled on the EKG.

3. D: When calculating the duration and amplitude on an EKG, values are typically reported to the nearest 0.5 mm or hundredth of a sec if they are slightly above or below or before or beyond a box unless detailed precision is critical. In this case, the duration of the P wave is 0.12 sec (three small boxes, $0.04 \times 3 = 0.12$), the amplitude is 2 mm (two small boxes, $1 \text{ mm} \times 2 = 2 \text{ mm}$), and the appearance is notched.

4. C: Somatic tremor artifacts are the result of involuntary muscle movements, which may occur if the patient is cold and shivering or has a condition that causes tremors, such as Parkinson's disease. Somatic tremor artifacts are characterized by rapid, repetitive, and erratic baseline fluctuations that have no consistent pattern and can be found in all leads; however, they are usually more evident in limb leads. Somatic tremor artifacts may be mistaken for atrial fibrillation.

5. C: The normal average body temperature in humans is 98.6 degrees Fahrenheit or 37 degrees Celsius.

6. C: The preferred site to take a pulse rate in pediatric patients 5 years or younger is the apical pulse.

7. C: Because the heart rate is regular, either the R-R method or the sequencing method can be used to calculate the heart rate.

- R-R method (count the number of small boxes between the R-R): 6 large boxes between R-R = 30 small boxes. 1,500/30 = 50 bpm.
- Sequencing method (memorize the sequence or refer to a chart): 6 large boxes = 50 bpm.

8. B: The EKG strip shows left atrial enlargement. This is a common finding with mitral stenosis. Lead II P-wave findings:

- Normal: <0.12 sec width and <2.5 mm amplitude
- Right atrial enlargement: Width unchanged but amplitude >2.5 mm; may be notched
- Left atrial enlargement: Amplitude unchanged but duration >0.12 sec; may be notched
- Right and left atrial enlargement: Both width and amplitude increased

9. D: The definition of supine is lying on the back with the face upward. Prone is the position of lying on the stomach with the head turned to one side. Dorsal refers to the back of the body. Prostrate is defined as being stretched out, face-down.

10. A, C, D: The speed of the EKG may be changed from 25 mm/s to 50 mm/s for EKG exams on infants and young children because their heart rates are typically much faster than those of adults. Additionally, if the heart rate is rapid because of SVT or atrial fibrillation with a rapid ventricular response, stretching the waveform may make it easier to analyze the P waves and QRS complex. If it is difficult to distinguish between P and T waves, such as with atrial flutter, the 50 mm/s speed may make them easier to distinguish.

11. D: The Occupational Safety and Health Administration's (OSHA's) job is to ensure safety in the workplace. It requires the employer to provide free, functioning safety gear, open disclosure about potential work hazards, and a system of reporting lapses in safety. OSHA does not address job benefits and vacation time.

12. C: Endocarditis, or the presence of vegetation(s) on a heart valve, can be diagnosed with direct visualization on a transthoracic echo or a transesophageal echo. An EKG is not a diagnostic test for endocarditis.

13. B: Ignoring someone who is doing something illegal, unethical, or immoral is not appropriate. The action should be addressed by someone. It is reasonable to confront the person yourself. It is equally reasonable to go directly to a supervisor and have them address the issue. In this case, since the medical records were not properly disposed of, they should be removed from the trash can and be placed in a proper hospital-designated trash receptacle.

14. C: If a patient has an implanted cardiac monitor, the electrodes should be placed to the side of the implant. In this case, the electrode should be placed to the left of the usual V2 position. Electrodes should not be placed over an implanted cardiac monitor because this can interfere with the device's ability to detect heart rhythms; may cause electrical interference with the EKG signal; and may, in rare circumstances, interfere with the functioning of the device.

15. C: Right bundle branch block occurs when the electrical impulse through the right bundle branch is delayed or blocked so that the right ventricle depolarizes later than the left ventricle. This delay results in an M appearance of the QRS complex in lead V1 and a W appearance in lead V6. Because the depolarization of the right ventricle is delayed, the QRS complex is typically widened to greater than 0.12 sec. The T waves are inverted in leads V1 through V3.

16. A: Of the choices for EKG leads given, response A describes the bipolar or standard limb leads, response B describes the augmented leads, and response D describes the chest or precordial leads.

17. B: Second-degree type I heart block (Mobitz type I) is characterized by normal-appearing P waves and a normal QRS complex (<0.12 sec), but there is a gradual prolonging of the P-R intervals with the distance lengthening between the P wave and the QRS complex until the QRS complex is dropped. The cycle then repeats. While the atrial rate is generally normal with a regular rhythm, the ventricular rate is slower because of the dropped QRS complexes and is irregular.

18. D: Manufacturing guidelines may vary somewhat, but generally the minimum safe distance between the pacemaker and the recorder is 6 inches. Most modern pacemakers have shielding against external electrical interference, although, if a Holter monitor with wireless telemetry is placed too close to a pacemaker, the pacemaker may misinterpret the electrical signals. The bigger concern is that the pacemaker will interfere with the Holter monitor, which can cause the monitor to pick up pacemaker signals rather than actual heart activity, misinterpret the pacing spikes, distort real EKG changes, or corrupt data. Some monitors have pacemaker-friendly settings.

19. C: The Lewis lead EKG modification is typically done to enhance detection of atrial activity or hidden P waves. It may also be used to assess wide complex tachycardia. Various configurations may be used; however, it is common to place the RA electrode on the manubrium, the LA electrode over the fifth intercostal space at the right sternal line, the RL electrode on the RL (standard position), and the LL electrode over the right lower costal margin.

20. B: A question that is designed to prompt only a yes or no response is a closed question. An open-ended question is one designed to prompt more information and therefore facilitate therapeutic communication. An indirect statement, which can also encourage therapeutic communication, is posed in a form such as "Tell me about..." Active listening is a good way of observing what a patient is communicating nonverbally.

21. A: Infants younger than 2 years old require right-sided placement of EKG electrodes (i.e., the same position as for dextrocardia) because the heart in neonates and infants is positioned more toward the right and midline. As the infant grows, the heart position shifts toward the left. In young infants, the right ventricle also tends to be dominant and the right-sided EKG is more likely to detect congenital heart conditions. Appropriately sized electrodes should always be used for neonates and infants. A 3-lead EKG is also commonly used instead of a 12-lead.

22. B: Patients with implanted cardiac pacemakers may go into cardiac arrest and can be defibrillated, but the defibrillator paddles should be at least 5 inches away from the pacemaker's battery pack. Defibrillators deliver a high-voltage shock that can disrupt pacemaker function or trigger inappropriate pacing or inhibition. Additionally, the shock may damage the pacemaker circuitry or partially dissipate into the pacemaker instead of the cardiac myocardium, resulting in incomplete defibrillation. If a paddle is too close to the battery pack, the shock may travel through the lead wires and cause localized damage to the heart.

23. D: Hepatitis C is an infection of the liver that is transmitted through sex, infected blood products, or contaminated needles. AIDS is also transmitted through the same mechanisms but dies quickly in the air. A medical provider is much more likely to get hepatitis C from a needle stick than AIDS. Roseola and varicella are viral infections that occur in childhood and are not transmitted through blood.

24. A: Universal precautions dictate that medical providers treat all patients and bodily fluids as if they had communicable diseases. Preventative measures such as gloves and consistent hand washing should be done at all times.

25. A: The calibration mark on the EKG tracing should be checked to ensure that the EKG machine is functioning properly and that the waveforms are accurately scaled. The calibration mark usually appears at the beginning of the tracing, and, if the EKG is taken at default speed with standard gain, it should be 10 mm (1 mV or two large squares) high and 5 mm (0.2 sec or five small boxes) wide.

The calibration marks ensure that the EKG is properly displaying electrical signals and standardizes EKGs so they can be compared among different settings and EKG machines. If the wave is abnormal, that indicates a problem.

26. C: Active listening requires the receiver to be attuned not only to what the other person is saying, but also to what they may be hinting at through body language or nonverbal communication. Being alert and interested is helpful but does not in itself constitute active listening. Maintaining eye contact can be helpful at times but is neither essential nor sufficient. Making a quick response defining a corrective action is generally thought to be detrimental to communication.

27. D: The precordial leads in a 12-lead EKG record electrical activity in the horizontal plane (anterior and posterior and right/left). The 6 precordial leads are placed on the chest, while the 6 limb leads are placed on the arms and legs and record electrical activity in the frontal plane (up and down and right/left). If necessary, arm electrodes can be positioned on the shoulders and leg electrodes can be positioned on the inferior rib cage without a significant change in signal.

28. A: Objective data is that which can be observed and measured in some way, such as a patient's blood pressure, heart rate, and respiration rate. Subjective observations should be recorded with objective descriptions. For example, if a patient appears confused, an appropriate documentation may be, "Patient is unable to recall birthdate or home address." This gives specific information that shows the patient's condition. In some cases, using direct quotations is a good choice. For example, instead of documenting, "Patient is upset about the wait time," a better description is, "Patient states, 'Waiting an hour for a visit is ridiculous.'"

29. A: The EKG changes that are common to myocardial injury and myocardial infarction include ST segment elevation and T-wave inversion, so onset of these changes should signal the need for further testing, such as cardiac enzymes and proteins. With myocardial ischemia, the first stage of heart damage, ST-segment depression and T-wave inversion are common. In the second stage, when the ischemia is prolonged and damage occurs, then ST-segment elevation is evident. In the third stage, myocardial infarction, the first change may be tall T-waves, but these become inverted and ST-segment elevation occurs as the hours pass.

30. A: Temperatures taken from within a body cavity are much more accurate than those taken from a body surface. Oral temperatures can be fairly accurate, but in some circumstances may not be able to be taken properly. An oral temperature may not be accurate if a patient is intubated or is a young child. In those cases, a rectal temperature is best.

31. D: HIPAA covers all of the issues discussed in choices A through C as well as a number of others, such as tax breaks for medical savings accounts, in its five titles. However, the only reference in HIPAA to Medicare type plans is that they must coordinate with other plans to prevent duplication of coverage.

32. B: If a patient has an implanted pacemaker, the location of the pacing spikes on the EKG depends on the type of pacing. Spikes typically are no more than 2 ms and may be difficult to detect in all leads. With atrial pacing, the pacing spike precedes the P wave. However, with ventricular pacing, the pacing spike precedes the QRS complex. With dual-chamber pacing, a pacing spike may appear before the P wave, before the QRS complex, or before both.

33. B: Individuals may vary depending on their general condition, but typically with every increase in the level of exertion during an exercise stress test, the patient's heart rate will increase by 10 bpm. If the heart rate increase is blunted, this may indicate autonomic dysfunction, a conduction disorder, or the use of medications to slow the heart, such as beta blockers. If the heart rate is excessively high, this may indicate deconditioning, anemia, or cardiac disorders, such as atrial tachycardia.

34. A: A living will is an advance directive. It usually names a power of attorney who is someone that will verbalize their wishes and can make medical decisions if the patient is unable to speak for him/herself. It also usually dictates the type of interventions the patient does or does not want. For example, a person may not want to be intubated, receive dialysis, or receive life-saving measures if they are not expected to have a full recovery.

35. A: Wide-complex pulsed VT and pulseless VT may appear identical on an EKG tracing. The primary difference is that with pulseless VT, the patient has no pulse and is unresponsive. Therefore, when this type of VT is observed, it is essential to assess the patient's level of consciousness and to ensure the patient has a pulse and respirations. Pulseless VT often rapidly changes into ventricular fibrillation. With VT, the rate is usually between 100 and 200.

36. C: With failure to capture, the heart does not respond with depolarization after a pacing spike. The EKG will show the pacing spike but without a corresponding P wave or QRS complex, resulting in bradycardia. Causes of failure to capture include lead displacement, fibrosis at the lead tip, battery depletion, circuit malfunction, hyperkalemia, hypermagnesemia, cardiac ischemia, and myocardial infarct. Inappropriate pacemaker programming, such as an output setting that is too low or the incorrect pacing mode, may also result in failure to capture.

37. B: Modified Mason-Likar EKG electrode placement involves placing the limb leads on the upper chest and lower torso rather than on the limbs. The LL electrode is placed in the lower left abdominal quadrant, and the RL electrode is placed in the lower right abdominal quadrant. This configuration is often used for patients with Parkinson's disease or other types of tremors to reduce artifacts associated with tremors. Precordial leads V1 through V6 are placed in their standard positions.

38. A: This EKG strip represents sinus tachycardia, which is characterized by regular atrial and ventricular rates and a heart rate between 100 and 160 bpm. The P wave is usually normal in size and shape and occurs before each QRS complex, although the amplitude may be increased. If the heart rate is too rapid, the P wave may be difficult to identify or may be superimposed on the preceding T wave. While the Q-T interval usually shortens, the P-R interval, QRS complex, and T wave are typically normal.

39. B: Torsades de pointes is characterized by a rapid irregular heart rate (typically 150–250 bpm), absent P waves and P-R interval, and wide QRS complexes. The QRS complexes reverse polarity, and a spindle effect (i.e., a gradual increase and decrease in amplitude) is present. The QRS complex may appear to be twisting around the baseline. The QT interval is long. A patient with torsades de pointes may present either with a pulse or without a pulse.

40. D: Third-degree SA block appears the same as sinus arrest on the EKG; however, with sinus arrest, the SA node does not generate an impulse. With third-degree SA block, the SA node generates an impulse, but there is a failure of the impulse to exit the SA node and depolarize the atria, resulting in an absence of P waves. This will either trigger an escape rhythm on the EKG, or it will result in asystole.

41. D: A pulse oximeter (also known as a "pulse ox") can be placed on a finger, ear, or toe, and helps measure oxygen saturation. It is usually seen on telemetry floors and in the intensive care unit.

42. D: V1 normally has a small R wave that gets progressively larger toward V6, so if the R wave in V1 is larger than in V2, the EKG technician should suspect that V1 and V2 are reversed. Additionally, V1 should show that the QRS complex is primarily negative, so if the QRS is primarily positive, this also suggests reversal. If reversal is not detected, the EKG interpretation may indicate a myocardial infarction, right ventricular hypertrophy, or a bundle branch block.

43. C: The Zio XT patch monitor is placed in the left upper chest. The top of the adhesive label should be one finger length below the clavicle (this puts the device itself two finger lengths below the clavicle). The area on the top label should be pointing upward, and the edge of the label is lined up along the edge of the left sternum. This positions the device in the center of the left pectoral muscle on the flattened area of the upper chest.

44. C: Second-degree heart block (Mobitz type II) is a type of heart block in which intermittent, nonconducted P waves result in a missing QRS complex, but the PR interval in conducted beats is usually constant but may be prolonged, and the P waves appear at the expected rate. This type of heart block is usually the result of conduction failure in the bundle of His (20%) or the Purkinje fibers (80%).

45. C: The Q-T interval extends from the beginning of the QRS complex to the end of the T wave. The normal duration of the Q-T interval is ≤0.44 sec for men and ≤0.46 sec for women. In this case, there are three large boxes comprising the Q-T interval, which is equal to 0.60 sec ($0.20 \times 3 = 0.60$ sec). A prolonged Q-T interval may be congenital or acquired. T wave abnormalities (broad, notched, biphasic) are also usually present. A prolonged Q-T interval increases the risk of life-threatening arrhythmias, such as torsades de pointes.

46. B: Patients with cardiovascular or respiratory problems should be positioned in either the semi-Fowler's or high Fowler's position, which are at 45- and 90-degree angles sitting up, respectively, to help them breathe. The dorsal recumbent or lithotomy position has patients lie on their back with their knees flexed and their feet either on the table or in attached stirrups. This position is used for genital and pelvic examinations, urinary catheterization, and other examinations. The Trendelenburg position has patients lie supine on their back with their feet elevated. This position is used to increase blood flow to the brain in emergencies and during abdominal or pelvic surgery. The Sims' position has patients lie laterally on their left side. This position is used for situations like vaginal and rectal exams, sigmoidoscopy, etc.

47. A: Weather is an external barrier to communication, as it may cause a distraction that draws the listener or speaker's attention away from the message being sent. Internal barriers are issues or problems that are occurring within the person such as stress, anger, hunger, depression, or pain. These issues can affect concentration and mental processes.

48. B: A normal heart rate in an adult human is 60–100 beats per minute. Those who are elderly, in excellent physical condition, or sleeping may have lower heart rates. Conditions such as stress, exercise, thyroid dysfunctions, or illness may cause an elevated heart rate.

49. B: If a patient is in late-term pregnancy, the enlarged uterus can press on the inferior vena cava if the patient lies in supine position, which can reduce the flow of blood to the heart and cause hypotension and dizziness as well as fetal distress. The patient should be placed in left lateral tilt position with a pillow under her right side to maintain the tilt. If the patient cannot tolerate this position, then a low semi-Fowler's position can be used.

50. B: A normal respiratory rate in a healthy adult is 12–20 breaths per minute. Below this range is called bradypnea, and above this range is called tachypnea.

51. B: CPR, or cardiopulmonary resuscitation, is indicated when an individual is found unresponsive and pulseless (or with a dangerously low pulse). Per AHA guidelines, CPR should be initiated as quickly as possible for maximum effect, starting with chest compressions. For circulation, 30 chest compressions should be administered rapidly, at a depth of 2" to 2.5", followed by 2 rescue breaths, with this cycle repeating until help has arrived and/or the defibrillator has been applied, charged, and is prepared to deliver a shock.

52. D: Standard precautions are a set of medical practice guidelines that are meant to protect healthcare workers from infection. Healthcare workers are instructed to use standard precautions to prevent contact with blood and all other potentially infectious substances. In any situation where there may be exposure to bodily fluids (e.g., blood, cerebral spinal fluid, vaginal secretions), employees should wear personal protective equipment (e.g., gloves, masks, gowns, and eye protection) and wash their hands. These guidelines apply to the care of all patients, regardless of status.

53. C: An echocardiogram uses ultrasound to assess the structure and function of the heart. However, three or four electrodes are placed to monitor the heart rhythm and synchronize the images with the heart's electrical activity. Once the electrodes are in place, the patient is placed in left lateral decubitus position. Electrodes typically used include RA (near the right clavicle), LA (near the left clavicle), and LL (on the lower right or left chest or abdomen). The LL electrode is often placed on the right so that it does not interfere with the ultrasound transducer. The RL electrode may be added as a ground electrode.

54. C: The sequencing method of determining the heart rate requires memorization of a sequence of numbers based on the numbers of small or large boxes between R waves. The corresponding boxes and heart rates using this method are as follows:

Small squares	Large squares	Bpm
5	1	300
10	2	150
15	3	100
20	4	75
25	5	60
30	6	50
35	7	43
40	8	37

Thus, if there are 25 small boxes (5 large boxes) between R waves, the pulse is 60.

55. A: A normal QRS is 0.08–0.012 seconds or two to three small boxes on an EKG.

56. C: If an employee is accidentally exposed to blood or other potentially infectious materials, they should be tested for HBV, HCV, and HIV (assuming they consent to the test) and offered prophylaxis if a test is positive. The employer must offer the employee a confidential medical evaluation, but the employee has the right to refuse this as well. The incident must be immediately reported to a superior and documented. Additional requirements include testing of the source blood if the patient consents, counseling of the employee, and submission of an OSHA 301 form.

57. B: The Q-T interval extends from the beginning of the Q deflection to the end of the T wave and represents the total time for ventricular depolarization and repolarization. In the tracing, the Q-T interval is 0.48 sec or 480 ms.

- Each large box is equal to 0.20 seconds: 0.20 × 2 = 0.40 sec.
- Each small box in the remaining box is equal to 0.04 sec: 0.04 × 2 = 0.08 sec.
- 0.40 + 0.08 = 0.48 sec, or 480 ms.

58. C: A person with a blood pressure of 165/81 mm Hg has hypertension. Hypertension is the medical term for elevated blood pressure. A normal blood pressure for an adult is 120/80 mm Hg. A single elevated blood pressure is not diagnostic of hypertension. There should be several consecutive pressures taken (usually 3 consecutive times spaced a few weeks apart) in order to be given this diagnosis.

59. C: Shockable rhythms include ventricular fibrillation and pulseless ventricular tachycardia (VT), which is characterized by a rapid heart rate of >100 bpm that originates from the ventricles. Because the heart rate is so rapid, the ventricles are unable to adequately fill, so the heart cannot pump blood effectively. The systolic BP falls to <80, and a pulse cannot be detected. The EKG tracing may show a narrow or wide QRS complex. If untreated, the patient will lose consciousness.

60. D: The P wave represents atrial depolarization, which is initiated by the SA node. The isoelectric line following the P wave indicates a delay at the AV node to prevent simultaneous atrial and ventricular contractions. Atrial repolarization is hidden in the QRS complex, which represents ventricular depolarization. The isoelectric line that follows the QRS complex indicates that depolarization is complete and represents ventricular repolarization, which begins at the heart apex. The T wave represents ventricular repolarization. The isoelectric line that follows the T wave indicates that repolarization is complete.

61. B: The P wave represents atrial depolarization during which the electrical activity spreads through the atria, causing the atria to contract. The valves separating the atria from the ventricles open, and most of the blood easily flows into the ventricles with the last 30% being pushed by the atrial contraction. Depolarization occurs first in the right atrium because this is the location of the SA node. Then, it spreads to the left atrium by Bachmann's bundle and then moves toward the AV node.

62. B: Before the patient can be shocked with the defibrillator, the electrodes that were in place for the EKG must be removed, so the EKG technician should do that immediately. Electrodes can create a barrier that prevents the AED pads from making direct skin contact. Additionally, the electrodes may cause electrical artifacts that can interfere with rhythm interpretation, and the electrical current may arc between metal parts of the EKG electrodes and increase the risk of burns.

63. B: Failure to sense may result in over- or undersensing and occurs when the pacemaker is unable to detect intrinsic cardiac activity, resulting in pacing randomly at inappropriate times. The pacing spike, for example, may occur within the QRS complex. If the spike occurs within the T wave, this can result in R-on-T arrhythmias, which can lead to ventricular fibrillation or VT. Failure to sense can be caused by lead displacement, depleted battery, incorrect sensitivity settings, and myocardial infarction.

64. D: ST segment depression occurs when the ST segment is at least 0.5 mm (0.05 mV) below the isoelectric line in ≥ contiguous leads. The depression may be downsloping, horizontal, or upsloping, depending on the underlying cause. Upsloping ST depression is typically the least concerning. ST

168

segment depression may indicate myocardial ischemia, non-ST elevation myocardial infarction, posterior myocardial infarction, bundle branch block, left ventricular hypertrophy, electrolyte imbalance, or digoxin effect.

65. B: All of the given choices are types of torts, which are wrongful actions that culminate in injury to the other person (in this case, the patient). Battery is the touching of a patient in a manner to which they have not consented. Invasion of privacy includes a number of situations in which a patient's privacy is invaded, such as releasing information about them without permission or failing to shield them properly during examination. Libel and slander are two types of defamation of character: false and malicious writing or speaking about someone, respectively.

66. B: Dextrocardia, a congenital condition in which the heart is located in the right chest, may be isolated with the other organs in their normal positions or mirrored with other organs also in opposite positions. For an EKG, the V1 and V2 electrodes are placed on opposite sides for the standard EKG with V1 at the fourth intercostal space to the left of the sternum and V2 to the right. The other chest electrodes are placed on the right chest in positions that mirror left-sided heart placement.

67. B: To reduce the risk of falls, the upper siderails of a bed are typically raised and the lower siderails are kept down so the patient can sit on the side of the bed or get out of bed. When administering an EKG for a patient, the upper siderail on the side that the EKG technician is working can be lowered while the technician applies the electrodes, but once the electrodes are in place, then the siderail should be raised again. Patients should never be left unattended with the upper siderails lowered.

68. D: If a patient has scars on the chest, such as from a left total mastectomy, and the scars extend over the usual V2 to V6 electrode positions, the electrodes should be placed below the scar in approximate positions and not on the scar tissue itself. In some cases, if scarring is severe and electrode placement in the chest is impossible or limited so that a clear signal cannot be obtained, posterior EKG leads V7–V9 may be considered.

69. B: Different types of technology can be used for telemetry:

- Radiofrequency: Have a typical range of 300–1,000 feet, depending on the setup, and they operate in the 400–600 MHz range to allow for better penetration of walls. This is the most common system in use. Examples include the GE ApexPro and Philips IntelliVue.
- Wi-Fi: Have a typical range throughout the facility and across hospital networks.
- Bluetooth: Have a typical range of 30–100 feet so they are most often used for outpatient monitoring, such as within the home, than for hospital telemetry.

70. B, C, E: The EKG technician must be alert to changes in cardiac rhythm during testing and must call for help immediately if potentially lethal dysrhythmias occur because any delay could result in the patient's death. Potentially lethal dysrhythmias are those that can lead to cardiac arrest or hemodynamic collapse and do not produce adequate cardiac output to sustain life. Potentially lethal dysrhythmias include VT, ventricular fibrillation, third-degree heart block, agonal rhythm, asystole, and pulseless electrical activity.

71. D: HIPAA (Health Insurance Portability and Accountability Act) requires that all employees of a medical facility maintain patient confidentiality, no matter what role they play in the patient's care.

72. D: Keeping one's voice low would not help facilitate communication in an elderly patient. Most elderly patients have hearing difficulties. When speaking to the elderly, one should speak in a loud, clear, slow voice so that no information is missed.

73. A: A pulse oximeter is a medical device that indirectly monitors the oxygen saturation of a patient's blood. A normal reading should be 94–100 percent. Patients with chronic obstructive pulmonary disease or pneumonia may have lower readings. A pulse ox of 75 percent would require intubation and mechanical ventilation. A pulse ox of 50 percent is not consistent with life.

74. D: Calipers are often used to more accurately interpret an EKG tracing, especially to measure the regularity of the rhythms. For example, one caliper point is on an R wave and the other caliper point is on the following R wave; then, this caliper setting is used to assess the following R-R intervals to determine if they are equal in duration. Calipers may also be used to measure the P-P interval, P-R interval, QRS duration, and QT interval.

75. D: The five-lead EKG requires five electrodes and can actually display six or more leads (I, II, III, aVR, aVL, aVF, and the precordial lead):

- RA (right arm)—white: Placed below the clavicle at the midclavicular line
- LA (left arm)—black: Placed below the clavicle at the midclavicular line
- RL (right leg)—green: Placed at the right lower abdomen
- LL (left leg)—red: Placed at the left lower abdomen
- V (chest lead)—brown: Usually placed at V1; may be moved to other positions (Ve–V6) for specific monitoring needs

76. D: While manufacturers' instructions may vary, telemetry alarms are commonly classified and set according to the severity of the problem and risk to the patient:

- High priority (life-threatening): Ventricular fibrillation, asystole, severe bradycardia (<30 bpm), severe prolonged tachycardia, third-degree atrioventricular (AV) heart block, ST elevation
- Medium priority (concerning): Premature atrial contractions, frequent premature ventricular contractions (PVCs), tachycardia (short run, not prolonged), atrial fibrillation (new onset), ST depression, a sudden drop in the heart rate, second-degree AV heart block,
- Low priority: Electrode off, motion artifact, infrequent PVCs, stable sinus tachycardia (100–130 bpm)

77. C: Tone of voice is a type of verbal communication. Gestures, posture, facial expression, proximity, and eye contact are all nonverbal types of communication.

78. D: Response C applies to CDC recommendations for use of Standard Precautions, but the OSHA Bloodborne Pathogens Standard goes further to include the items in response D.

79. C: A person who is chronically homeless is likely very hungry. This kind of internal barrier may affect effective communication. Internal barriers are issues or problems that are occurring within the person such as stress, anger, hunger, depression, or pain. These issues can affect concentration and mental processes.

80. D: The history of present illness (HPI) includes subjective information that the patient gives to the medical practitioner such as chief complaint, associated symptoms, pain quality, and scale. The HPI also includes past medical history, past surgical history, social history, family history, allergies, and medications. The physical exam contains objective findings seen by the medical professional.

81. B: Zone 2.

Zone	% of MHR	Intensity	Rate of Perceived Exertion
1	50–60	Very light	Very easy (e.g., gentle walking, stretching)
2	60–70	Light	Comfortable and able to speak easily (e.g., brisk walking, swimming)
3	70–80	Moderate	Challenging but able to sustain, can still speak (e.g., running, steady cycling)
4	80–90	Hard	Breathing hard, only able to speak in short sentences (e.g., fast cycling, stair climbing)
5	90–100	Maximum	Maximum effort, unsustainable, difficulty trying to speak (e.g., sprinting, high-intensity interval training)

82. D: A patient who is passed out and unconscious but has a pulse and normal respirations should be placed in the lateral recumbent "recovery" position to maintain an open airway and prevent aspiration. The patient is rolled onto the side with the top knee in contact with the floor or other surface in order to support the body. The patient's hand is placed under the head to maintain the head in a neutral position.

83. B: An escape rhythm is one that is generated outside of the SA node as a backup when normal transmission of an electrical impulse fails. While the AV node (i.e., the primary pacemaker) normally generates impulses at the rate of 60–100 bpm, a junctional escape rhythm, which originates in the AV junction (i.e., the AV node and bundle of His), has an intrinsic rate of 40–60 bpm. On the EKG, the junctional escape rhythm is characterized by inverted, absent, or otherwise misplaced P waves; a narrow QRS complex; and a short P-R interval.

84. A: For emergency transport, a basic 3-lead EKG setup is typically used because it requires only three electrodes and is easy and fast to set up. While the 3-lead EKG is not used for diagnosis, it can detect life-threatening arrhythmias that may occur in emergency situations and can also detect patient response to medications or treatments administered during transit. Additionally, the 3-lead system is less sensitive to motion artifacts, and ambulances and air transportation are in constant motion.

85. B: When a patient is having a Holter monitor applied, the first thing to do is to check the batteries to ensure that they are fully charged and ready for use because weak batteries may interfere with the recording or may shut off the device. Different kinds of batteries are used, depending on the type of Holter monitor and the age of the monitor. Older monitors may use disposable alkaline or disposable or rechargeable lithium batteries. Newer and wireless Holter monitors use rechargeable lithium-ion or lithium polymer batteries, which are often charged with a USB cord or a docking station.

86. B: Ethics refers to the set of personal values that shape an individual's perceptions of right and wrong, which is different from morals. Ethics are not laws defining acceptable behavior or creeds to live by, although the latter generally are derived from ethics.

87. B: A blood pressure measurement in itself is written as "systolic pressure/diastolic pressure" (for example: 110/75), but it is preferable to also note the arm used and the patient position (for example: right arm, supine).

88. A: Monomorphic and polymorphic VT share similar characteristics: the heart rate usually ranges from 150–250 bpm, the P wave may be absent or not associated with the QRS complex, and the P-R interval is absent. However, while monomorphic VT typically has a regular rhythm, the rhythm for polymorphic VT may be regular or irregular. The most significant difference is that, with monomorphic VT, the QRS complexes are the same shape and amplitude but, with polymorphic VT, they vary in shape and amplitude.

89. D: The EKG tracing shown is an example of an elevated ST segment. The ST segment should be on or ≤1mm above or below the isoelectric line in the limb leads. In the precordial leads, an elevation of up to 2 mm may be normal in some individuals, but if the elevation is greater than 1 mm in limb leads or greater than 2 mm in precordial leads, this suggests acute myocardial infarction or other cardiac abnormality.

90. B: An EMR is an electronic medical record from a single source, such as a medical practice, but when EMRs from various sources are combined to generate a comprehensive electronic patient database, they constitute an EHR. MOSS is a type of TPMS.

91. D: The five-lead configuration for a Holter monitor typically includes:

- RA (white): Right upper chest, below the clavicle
- LA (black): Left upper chest, below the clavicle
- LL (red): Upper left abdomen
- RL (green): Upper right abdomen
- VI or C (brown): Fourth intercostal space, right of the sternum

For a seven-lead configuration, two additional electrodes are added:

- V3 (orange): Midway between the fourth intercostal space left of the sternum (V2 position) and the fifth intercostal space, midclavicular line (V4 position)
- V5 (purple): Left anterior axillary line, fifth intercostal space

92. B: Orthopnea, or labored breathing, is difficulty breathing unless standing or sitting erect; it occurs in conditions like angina pectoris, heart failure, and various pulmonary conditions. The other situations do involve a period of complete absence of breathing known as apnea. Sleep apnea is characterized by periods of more than 10 seconds in which breathing stops during sleep, depleting the brain of oxygen and potentially causing a variety of cardiac and neurologic defects. Cheyne-Stokes respiration is a respiration cycle in which there is approximately 10-60 seconds of apnea, then deep and rapid breathing, and then a decreased rate.

93. A: EKG strips are properly mounted in the same manner each time in vertical columns containing four strips:

Lead I	Lead II	Lead III
aVR	aVL	aVF
V1	V2	V3
V4	V3	V6

Standardizing mounting is important to avoid confusion so that everyone interprets the EKG the same way and follows the same sequence. Healthcare professionals, such as doctors and nurses, are trained to interpret EKG tracings using this standard EKG lead order. The strips should be carefully aligned, straight, and properly labeled and spaced.

94. B: EKG machines use two different types of paper, roll and Z-fold thermal paper. When loading a new supply of Z-fold thermal paper, first, check for any paper jams or remaining sheets from a previous stack and remove them so that the paper will feed smoothly. Z-fold thermal paper stacks do not need to be fanned or trimmed and should be loaded with the print side facing up so that it faces the print head. The paper should be properly aligned with the feed with one section extending out of the machine.

95. A: Anxiety can cause chest discomfort, but it is usually described as a sharp pain, and pain related to reflux is often burning. Hypertension may cause dizziness or headache, but not usually chest pain. Pressure in the chest is a classic sign of cardiac ischemia or heart attack (myocardial infarction). If this occurs, the EKG technician should immediately stop the test, call for help, assist the patient to a sitting or lying position, and check his or her vital signs.

96. C: A relaxed versus a rigid posture creates feelings of ease, trust, and serenity. Using a low voice in a reassuring tone helps contribute to that atmosphere. Maintaining consistent eye contact improves communication and helps build feelings of trust.

97. B: High peaked P waves in lead II are an indication of right atrial enlargement, most often due to pulmonary hypertension related to chronic respiratory disease, such as with patients with chronic obstructive pulmonary disease. The primary characteristic of tall, peaked P waves is an amplitude of ≥2.5 mm in lead II with a P wave duration of ≤0.12 sec (normal). Right atrial enlargement occurs when the right atrium dilates or hypertrophies because of increased pressure. This results in increased atrial electrical forces that produce the peaked P waves.

98. A: Steps to interpretation of an EKG:

- Analyze the rhythm (regular, irregular R-R intervals); the regularity of the rhythm will determine the best method to then determining the heart rate since irregular rhythms cannot be estimated in the same way that regular rhythms are.
- Determine the heart rate (normal: 60–100 bpm)
- Note the presence or absence of a P wave (normal: before each QRS complex and identical in size and shape)
- Measure the P-R interval (normal: 0.12–0.20 sec)
- Assess the QRS complex (normal: <0.12 sec)
- Evaluate the ST segment (normal: upright in most leads)
- Measure the Q-T interval (normal: <0.44 sec for men, and <0.46 sec for women)

99. B: Ethically and legally, it is your duty to protect your patients. If a colleague is coming to work while intoxicated, this could place patients at risk. You should report the situation to your supervisor so appropriate action can be taken. An intoxicated employee should not be working with patients.

100. B: The only one of these characteristics that distinguishes an electronic sphygmomanometer is that it does not necessitate simultaneous use of a stethoscope because there is a digital readout. There are three types of manometers, all of which use a pressure cuff: electronic, aneroid, and the traditional mercury type, which is being phased out. Response C is true of the aneroid type, which uses a dial attached to the rubber bladder pressure cuff.

How to Overcome Test Anxiety

Just the thought of taking a test is enough to make most people a little nervous. A test is an important event that can have a long-term impact on your future, so it's important to take it seriously and it's natural to feel anxious about performing well. But just because anxiety is normal, that doesn't mean that it's helpful in test taking, or that you should simply accept it as part of your life. Anxiety can have a variety of effects. These effects can be mild, like making you feel slightly nervous, or severe, like blocking your ability to focus or remember even a simple detail.

If you experience test anxiety—whether severe or mild—it's important to know how to beat it. To discover this, first you need to understand what causes test anxiety.

Causes of Test Anxiety

While we often think of anxiety as an uncontrollable emotional state, it can actually be caused by simple, practical things. One of the most common causes of test anxiety is that a person does not feel adequately prepared for their test. This feeling can be the result of many different issues such as poor study habits or lack of organization, but the most common culprit is time management. Starting to study too late, failing to organize your study time to cover all of the material, or being distracted while you study will mean that you're not well prepared for the test. This may lead to cramming the night before, which will cause you to be physically and mentally exhausted for the test. Poor time management also contributes to feelings of stress, fear, and hopelessness as you realize you are not well prepared but don't know what to do about it.

Other times, test anxiety is not related to your preparation for the test but comes from unresolved fear. This may be a past failure on a test, or poor performance on tests in general. It may come from comparing yourself to others who seem to be performing better or from the stress of living up to expectations. Anxiety may be driven by fears of the future—how failure on this test would affect your educational and career goals. These fears are often completely irrational, but they can still negatively impact your test performance.

Elements of Test Anxiety

As mentioned earlier, test anxiety is considered to be an emotional state, but it has physical and mental components as well. Sometimes you may not even realize that you are suffering from test anxiety until you notice the physical symptoms. These can include trembling hands, rapid heartbeat, sweating, nausea, and tense muscles. Extreme anxiety may lead to fainting or vomiting. Obviously, any of these symptoms can have a negative impact on testing. It is important to recognize them as soon as they begin to occur so that you can address the problem before it damages your performance.

The mental components of test anxiety include trouble focusing and inability to remember learned information. During a test, your mind is on high alert, which can help you recall information and stay focused for an extended period of time. However, anxiety interferes with your mind's natural processes, causing you to blank out, even on the questions you know well. The strain of testing during anxiety makes it difficult to stay focused, especially on a test that may take several hours. Extreme anxiety can take a huge mental toll, making it difficult not only to recall test information but even to understand the test questions or pull your thoughts together.

Effects of Test Anxiety

Test anxiety is like a disease—if left untreated, it will get progressively worse. Anxiety leads to poor performance, and this reinforces the feelings of fear and failure, which in turn lead to poor performances on subsequent tests. It can grow from a mild nervousness to a crippling condition. If allowed to progress, test anxiety can have a big impact on your schooling, and consequently on your future.

Test anxiety can spread to other parts of your life. Anxiety on tests can become anxiety in any stressful situation, and blanking on a test can turn into panicking in a job situation. But fortunately, you don't have to let anxiety rule your testing and determine your grades. There are a number of relatively simple steps you can take to move past anxiety and function normally on a test and in the rest of life.

Physical Steps for Beating Test Anxiety

While test anxiety is a serious problem, the good news is that it can be overcome. It doesn't have to control your ability to think and remember information. While it may take time, you can begin taking steps today to beat anxiety.

Just as your first hint that you may be struggling with anxiety comes from the physical symptoms, the first step to treating it is also physical. Rest is crucial for having a clear, strong mind. If you are tired, it is much easier to give in to anxiety. But if you establish good sleep habits, your body and mind will be ready to perform optimally, without the strain of exhaustion. Additionally, sleeping well helps you to retain information better, so you're more likely to recall the answers when you see the test questions.

Getting good sleep means more than going to bed on time. It's important to allow your brain time to relax. Take study breaks from time to time so it doesn't get overworked, and don't study right before bed. Take time to rest your mind before trying to rest your body, or you may find it difficult to fall asleep.

Along with sleep, other aspects of physical health are important in preparing for a test. Good nutrition is vital for good brain function. Sugary foods and drinks may give a burst of energy but this burst is followed by a crash, both physically and emotionally. Instead, fuel your body with protein and vitamin-rich foods.

Also, drink plenty of water. Dehydration can lead to headaches and exhaustion, especially if your brain is already under stress from the rigors of the test. Particularly if your test is a long one, drink water during the breaks. And if possible, take an energy-boosting snack to eat between sections.

Along with sleep and diet, a third important part of physical health is exercise. Maintaining a steady workout schedule is helpful, but even taking 5-minute study breaks to walk can help get your blood pumping faster and clear your head. Exercise also releases endorphins, which contribute to a positive feeling and can help combat test anxiety.

When you nurture your physical health, you are also contributing to your mental health. If your body is healthy, your mind is much more likely to be healthy as well. So take time to rest, nourish your body with healthy food and water, and get moving as much as possible. Taking these physical steps will make you stronger and more able to take the mental steps necessary to overcome test anxiety.

How to Overcome Test Anxiety

Mental Steps for Beating Test Anxiety

Working on the mental side of test anxiety can be more challenging, but as with the physical side, there are clear steps you can take to overcome it. As mentioned earlier, test anxiety often stems from lack of preparation, so the obvious solution is to prepare for the test. Effective studying may be the most important weapon you have for beating test anxiety, but you can and should employ several other mental tools to combat fear.

First, boost your confidence by reminding yourself of past success—tests or projects that you aced. If you're putting as much effort into preparing for this test as you did for those, there's no reason you should expect to fail here. Work hard to prepare; then trust your preparation.

Second, surround yourself with encouraging people. It can be helpful to find a study group, but be sure that the people you're around will encourage a positive attitude. If you spend time with others who are anxious or cynical, this will only contribute to your own anxiety. Look for others who are motivated to study hard from a desire to succeed, not from a fear of failure.

Third, reward yourself. A test is physically and mentally tiring, even without anxiety, and it can be helpful to have something to look forward to. Plan an activity following the test, regardless of the outcome, such as going to a movie or getting ice cream.

When you are taking the test, if you find yourself beginning to feel anxious, remind yourself that you know the material. Visualize successfully completing the test. Then take a few deep, relaxing breaths and return to it. Work through the questions carefully but with confidence, knowing that you are capable of succeeding.

Developing a healthy mental approach to test taking will also aid in other areas of life. Test anxiety affects more than just the actual test—it can be damaging to your mental health and even contribute to depression. It's important to beat test anxiety before it becomes a problem for more than testing.

Study Strategy

Being prepared for the test is necessary to combat anxiety, but what does being prepared look like? You may study for hours on end and still not feel prepared. What you need is a strategy for test prep. The next few pages outline our recommended steps to help you plan out and conquer the challenge of preparation.

STEP 1: SCOPE OUT THE TEST

Learn everything you can about the format (multiple choice, essay, etc.) and what will be on the test. Gather any study materials, course outlines, or sample exams that may be available. Not only will this help you to prepare, but knowing what to expect can help to alleviate test anxiety.

STEP 2: MAP OUT THE MATERIAL

Look through the textbook or study guide and make note of how many chapters or sections it has. Then divide these over the time you have. For example, if a book has 15 chapters and you have five days to study, you need to cover three chapters each day. Even better, if you have the time, leave an extra day at the end for overall review after you have gone through the material in depth.

If time is limited, you may need to prioritize the material. Look through it and make note of which sections you think you already have a good grasp on, and which need review. While you are studying, skim quickly through the familiar sections and take more time on the challenging parts.

Write out your plan so you don't get lost as you go. Having a written plan also helps you feel more in control of the study, so anxiety is less likely to arise from feeling overwhelmed at the amount to cover.

STEP 3: GATHER YOUR TOOLS

Decide what study method works best for you. Do you prefer to highlight in the book as you study and then go back over the highlighted portions? Or do you type out notes of the important information? Or is it helpful to make flashcards that you can carry with you? Assemble the pens, index cards, highlighters, post-it notes, and any other materials you may need so you won't be distracted by getting up to find things while you study.

If you're having a hard time retaining the information or organizing your notes, experiment with different methods. For example, try color-coding by subject with colored pens, highlighters, or post-it notes. If you learn better by hearing, try recording yourself reading your notes so you can listen while in the car, working out, or simply sitting at your desk. Ask a friend to quiz you from your flashcards, or try teaching someone the material to solidify it in your mind.

STEP 4: CREATE YOUR ENVIRONMENT

It's important to avoid distractions while you study. This includes both the obvious distractions like visitors and the subtle distractions like an uncomfortable chair (or a too-comfortable couch that makes you want to fall asleep). Set up the best study environment possible: good lighting and a comfortable work area. If background music helps you focus, you may want to turn it on, but otherwise keep the room quiet. If you are using a computer to take notes, be sure you don't have any other windows open, especially applications like social media, games, or anything else that could distract you. Silence your phone and turn off notifications. Be sure to keep water close by so you stay hydrated while you study (but avoid unhealthy drinks and snacks).

Also, take into account the best time of day to study. Are you freshest first thing in the morning? Try to set aside some time then to work through the material. Is your mind clearer in the afternoon or evening? Schedule your study session then. Another method is to study at the same time of day that you will take the test, so that your brain gets used to working on the material at that time and will be ready to focus at test time.

STEP 5: STUDY!

Once you have done all the study preparation, it's time to settle into the actual studying. Sit down, take a few moments to settle your mind so you can focus, and begin to follow your study plan. Don't give in to distractions or let yourself procrastinate. This is your time to prepare so you'll be ready to fearlessly approach the test. Make the most of the time and stay focused.

Of course, you don't want to burn out. If you study too long you may find that you're not retaining the information very well. Take regular study breaks. For example, taking five minutes out of every hour to walk briskly, breathing deeply and swinging your arms, can help your mind stay fresh.

As you get to the end of each chapter or section, it's a good idea to do a quick review. Remind yourself of what you learned and work on any difficult parts. When you feel that you've mastered the material, move on to the next part. At the end of your study session, briefly skim through your notes again.

But while review is helpful, cramming last minute is NOT. If at all possible, work ahead so that you won't need to fit all your study into the last day. Cramming overloads your brain with more information than it can process and retain, and your tired mind may struggle to recall even

How to Overcome Test Anxiety

previously learned information when it is overwhelmed with last-minute study. Also, the urgent nature of cramming and the stress placed on your brain contribute to anxiety. You'll be more likely to go to the test feeling unprepared and having trouble thinking clearly.

So don't cram, and don't stay up late before the test, even just to review your notes at a leisurely pace. Your brain needs rest more than it needs to go over the information again. In fact, plan to finish your studies by noon or early afternoon the day before the test. Give your brain the rest of the day to relax or focus on other things, and get a good night's sleep. Then you will be fresh for the test and better able to recall what you've studied.

STEP 6: TAKE A PRACTICE TEST

Many courses offer sample tests, either online or in the study materials. This is an excellent resource to check whether you have mastered the material, as well as to prepare for the test format and environment.

Check the test format ahead of time: the number of questions, the type (multiple choice, free response, etc.), and the time limit. Then create a plan for working through them. For example, if you have 30 minutes to take a 60-question test, your limit is 30 seconds per question. Spend less time on the questions you know well so that you can take more time on the difficult ones.

If you have time to take several practice tests, take the first one open book, with no time limit. Work through the questions at your own pace and make sure you fully understand them. Gradually work up to taking a test under test conditions: sit at a desk with all study materials put away and set a timer. Pace yourself to make sure you finish the test with time to spare and go back to check your answers if you have time.

After each test, check your answers. On the questions you missed, be sure you understand why you missed them. Did you misread the question (tests can use tricky wording)? Did you forget the information? Or was it something you hadn't learned? Go back and study any shaky areas that the practice tests reveal.

Taking these tests not only helps with your grade, but also aids in combating test anxiety. If you're already used to the test conditions, you're less likely to worry about it, and working through tests until you're scoring well gives you a confidence boost. Go through the practice tests until you feel comfortable, and then you can go into the test knowing that you're ready for it.

Test Tips

On test day, you should be confident, knowing that you've prepared well and are ready to answer the questions. But aside from preparation, there are several test day strategies you can employ to maximize your performance.

First, as stated before, get a good night's sleep the night before the test (and for several nights before that, if possible). Go into the test with a fresh, alert mind rather than staying up late to study.

Try not to change too much about your normal routine on the day of the test. It's important to eat a nutritious breakfast, but if you normally don't eat breakfast at all, consider eating just a protein bar. If you're a coffee drinker, go ahead and have your normal coffee. Just make sure you time it so that the caffeine doesn't wear off right in the middle of your test. Avoid sugary beverages, and drink enough water to stay hydrated but not so much that you need a restroom break 10 minutes into the test. If your test isn't first thing in the morning, consider going for a walk or doing a light workout before the test to get your blood flowing.

Allow yourself enough time to get ready, and leave for the test with plenty of time to spare so you won't have the anxiety of scrambling to arrive in time. Another reason to be early is to select a good seat. It's helpful to sit away from doors and windows, which can be distracting. Find a good seat, get out your supplies, and settle your mind before the test begins.

When the test begins, start by going over the instructions carefully, even if you already know what to expect. Make sure you avoid any careless mistakes by following the directions.

Then begin working through the questions, pacing yourself as you've practiced. If you're not sure on an answer, don't spend too much time on it, and don't let it shake your confidence. Either skip it and come back later, or eliminate as many wrong answers as possible and guess among the remaining ones. Don't dwell on these questions as you continue—put them out of your mind and focus on what lies ahead.

Be sure to read all of the answer choices, even if you're sure the first one is the right answer. Sometimes you'll find a better one if you keep reading. But don't second-guess yourself if you do immediately know the answer. Your gut instinct is usually right. Don't let test anxiety rob you of the information you know.

If you have time at the end of the test (and if the test format allows), go back and review your answers. Be cautious about changing any, since your first instinct tends to be correct, but make sure you didn't misread any of the questions or accidentally mark the wrong answer choice. Look over any you skipped and make an educated guess.

At the end, leave the test feeling confident. You've done your best, so don't waste time worrying about your performance or wishing you could change anything. Instead, celebrate the successful completion of this test. And finally, use this test to learn how to deal with anxiety even better next time.

Review Video: Test Anxiety
Visit mometrix.com/academy and enter code: 100340

Important Qualification

Not all anxiety is created equal. If your test anxiety is causing major issues in your life beyond the classroom or testing center, or if you are experiencing troubling physical symptoms related to your anxiety, it may be a sign of a serious physiological or psychological condition. If this sounds like your situation, we strongly encourage you to seek professional help.

How to Overcome Test Anxiety

Online Resources

Due to our efforts to try to keep this book to a manageable length, we've created a link that will give you access to all of your online resources:

mometrix.com/resources719/nhaekgtech

It's Your Moment, Let's Celebrate It!

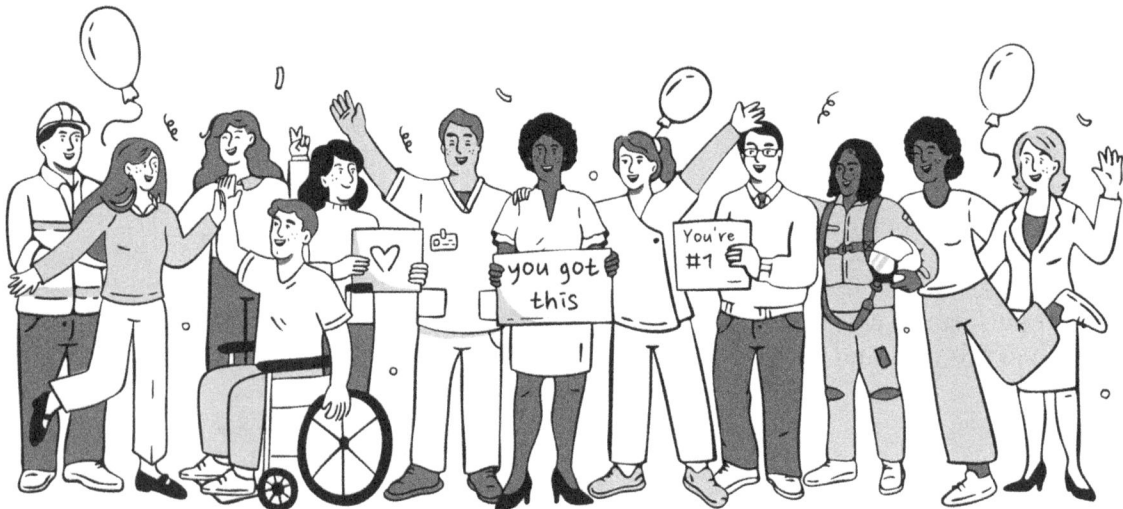

Share your story @mometrixtestpreparation

Made in the USA
Coppell, TX
26 June 2025

51133329R00105